BECAUSE

WE ARE BAD

OCD and a Girl Lost in Thought

LILY

BAILEY

Canbury Press

Published by Canbury Press, 2016

This edition published 2018

Canbury Press,

Kingston upon Thames, Surrey

www.canburypress.com

Cover: Tom Sanderson

Printed and bound in Great Britain by Clays Ltd, St Ives Plc

This is a work of non-fiction.

The events and experiences detailed herein are all true and have been faithfully rendered as I have remembered them, to the best of my ability. Some names, identities, and circumstances have been changed in order to protect the integrity and/or anonymity of the individuals concerned.

Though conversations come from my keen recollection of them, they are not written to represent word for word documentation; rather, I've retold them in a way that evokes the real feeling and meaning of what was said. In some cases, composite characters have been created or timelines have been compressed in order to further preserve privacy and to maintain narrative flow. This book does not contain any health advice.

Further information on OCD:

www.ocdaction.org.uk / www.ocduk.org

ISBN: 978-0-9930407-4-0 PB

978-0-9930407-2-6 HB

978-0-9930407-3-3 Ebook

Audiobook Available

For you,
you know who you are

CONTENTS

1. Chesbury Hospital 5

2. My Friend 7

3. The Letter 9

4. New School 14

5. Mum and Dad 22

6. Swearing in Church 31

7. Most Apologetic Girl 39

8. Hambledon 49

9. Running from Words 57

10. Stumbling 62

11. Special Needs Department 67

12. Coming Home 74

13. Doctor, Doctor 85

14. Pills, Pills, Pills 94

15. Driving 104

16. Those Who Love Me 118

17. Thailand 126

18. Dublin 141

19. It Is My Fault 157

20. Mental Ward 160

21. Harley Street 165

22. Urine Test 176

23. Loser, Friend 189

24. Skating 197

25. Ashleaves 204

26. Nursery 215

27. Journalism 227

28. Rocky 239

29. The Truth 248

1

Chesbury Hospital

From the outside, Chesbury Hospital in London looks like a castle that got lost and was plonked down in the wrong place. It is long and white, with battlements and arched windows from which princesses could call down, in the chapter before they are saved.

But it's not entirely believable. Where the portcullis should be, there are giant glass doors. Walk through them, and you could be in a five-star hotel. The man at reception wears a suit and tie and asks if he can help, like he's going to book you a table. A glass cupboard showcases the gifts sold by reception: bath oils, rejuvenating face cream, and Green & Black's chocolate, just in case you arrive empty-handed to see a crazy relative and need an icebreaker.

The walls, lampshades, window fittings, and radiators are all a similar, unnameable colour, somewhere between brown, yellow, and cream. A looping gold chandelier is suspended by a heavy chain; the fireplace has marble columns. The members of staff have busy, preoccupied faces—until they come close to you, when their mouths break into wide, fixed smiles.

Compared with the Harley Street clinic, there is a superior

choice of herbal teas. When the police arrived after the escape, Mum cried a lot; then she shouted. Now she has assumed a sense of British resolve. She queries: 'Wild Jasmine, Purple Rose, or Earl Grey?'

A nurse checks through my bag, which has been lugged upstairs. She takes the razor (fair enough), tweezers (sort of fair enough), a bottle of Baileys lying forgotten in the handbag (definitely fair enough), and headphones (definitely not fair enough). There would never be a hanging: far too much mess.

The observation room is next to the nurses' station; they keep you there until you are no longer a risk to yourself.

It is 10th January, 2013, and I am 19.

2

My Friend

In the playground, fads come and go consistently, without apparent supervision, like waves on a beach. We had Pokémon, we had Furbies; we had aliens encased in strange plastic eggs. Then at some point, when we were five, imaginary friends took off as a craze. People would save spaces at the lunch table for someone no one else could see. Girls would sit on the climbing frame, plaiting hair that looked like air to those without an imagination.

No one wanted to be that—a child without an imagination. It made you no fun to play with. It meant you got excluded from certain games. Some of those who said they had imaginary friends didn't really have any specific vision of what this friend might be like, nor did they really care for the craze at all. Desperately dull girls like Claudia couldn't even make up a good story when playing with a doll's house; how could they conjure up a whole person?

Some of the die-hard fans, the revolutionaries with sparky minds and endless originality, may have taken their imaginary friends home for dinner, shared a bath with them, and read them bedtime stories. But the majority were probably scattered somewhere between the two extremes. They could imagine something, if not necessarily a fully formed person, but when school ended, that was that. The friend was left behind at the gates, without a thought, until the next morning, when the craze demanded that she reappear. That was why this fad was terrifying; amid a constant onslaught of daily change and childhood adaptation, one thing had stayed weirdly constant in my life. For as long as I could remember, I wasn't me, I was we.

Two of us sat side by side in my head, woven together, inseparable. She didn't even have a name; she was just She. Really, it was hard to say where She ended and I began. But food was not shared with her. She did not play tag and never required a seat. She was, by her very essence, nothing like these imaginary friends. She was just there.

One was not proud of her, in the same way as one is not proud of a liver, and there was no need to show her off, nor tell anyone She existed.

But though her differences were concerning (why did other kids insist on parading their friends around? Were they just for show? Couldn't they see it didn't have to be a competition?), they were nothing compared to the fad's main implication. Because a fad demands that something that wasn't there before come into existence; and that meant only one thing. Normal children didn't have two people in their heads.

Which meant I must be very different, for mine was not the sort of friend to be left behind at the gates.

3

The Letter

It's home time. We are sitting in a circle in the classroom, and Miss Watts is putting a letter in our schoolbag. We wonder if it is a report. We have heard from the big kids in Year 2 that you get a report at the end of each term where the teacher writes about your progress.

Suddenly we are scared. The thought comes into our head that we have done something very bad this term, something we don't even remember doing, and that Miss Watts is about to tell Mum and Dad.

We go outside into the playground, clutching our schoolbag. Grandma Muriel is waiting to pick us up, as Mum and Dad are always at work, and our au pair has the day off. Grandma has crazy orange hair and huge glasses, and she folds us into a big warm hug. Our nostrils fill with the smell of Persil and cooking.

'Hello, my love! Do you want me to take your schoolbag?' she asks. We pull it close to our chest, afraid she will take it and tear open the report right here.

What is this bad thing we may have done this term? Perhaps we hit another child, or bit someone. Maybe we called someone names or said a rude word to a teacher. The pictures of these things happening become so real in our head, we are sure that we must have done them—they must be half-memories of the real thing happening.

'What's wrong with you?' says Grandma. 'You don't look yourself.'

We give her a big smile. 'I'm fine.'

Once we get home, we wait for Grandma to go to the toilet. Quickly, we dig the letter out of our bag and put it in the bin, pushing it right to the bottom and piling the rubbish on top of it. For a few seconds, we feel calm. We can still hear some sort of roaring in the side of our head, though it is softer now, like the sea when you hear it though a shell.

But what if Grandma knows what we have done and tries to retrieve the letter? That can't happen. The roaring gets louder; it sounds like the real sea, frothy and raging—as if it wants something.

For the next few hours we stand by the bin, offering to help Grandma whenever she needs to put in vegetable peel and other stuff. Grandma laughs. She says we remind her of the bin monitor she used to have at school.

'Grandma, what day do the bin men come?'

'Wednesday, I think.'

'What day is today?'

'Tuesday.'

'What time do they come?'

'In the morning. Early. You'd probably be asleep.'

'This bin bag needs to go outside.'

'It's not full yet.'

'Yes, it is. I need to put it outside.'

'Why this sudden fascination with bins, Lily? Okay, just to show you one time how it works, we'll put the bin bag outside together.'

We and Grandma haul the bin bag outside the front door. We're not really carrying much of the weight, but we still clutch the side of it to make sure Grandma doesn't run off with it. She tells us to lift the plastic lid off one of the big black bins, and we dump the bag inside. We feel better knowing the report is in the bin, but we won't feel truly safe until we know it's gone for good.

The next morning, we wake up very early. It's pitch-black outside. We creep into the spare room, which looks out on the bins. We will stay here until the bin men come—we will make sure that letter is gone for good.

It feels like it takes hours, but we don't think it can be that long. We hear it before we see it: a distant rumble getting closer. Then the lorry turns into our road. Giant and green with flashing lights, it crawls towards us a few doors at a time. Finally, it stops outside. Three men get out, and each takes a bag from the large black buckets. An old tall man with a beard takes the bag from the second bin—our bag. We watch him fling it into the back of the truck. Then they all get back in and drive on. We stay watching until the truck has well and truly disappeared.

The letter is gone now.

It will never hurt us. Everything is okay.

Our parents have been arguing about what type of school we should be at. There's a school round the corner where the kids wear a uniform and a straw hat. Sophie, who is in our class, calls it the Posh School, and you have to pay money to go there. It seems like we might be going to the Posh School, because although we didn't used to have much money, Dad has made some now.

Dad thinks it's a good idea to get us away from 'those girls.' But Mum doesn't agree because she doesn't want us to be snotty, and she doesn't think we'll get on with the crowd there. Dad says she needs to think about 'what is best for Lily.'

'They don't like her,' he hisses. 'The girls there. They're horrible to her. You saw—on her birthday, when we took them to the park. They just ran off and ignored her. She spent the whole time with us. She looked so sad. Don't you want her to have friends?'

We can't talk to them about this, because we're not even supposed to know. We heard about it a few nights ago when we couldn't sleep. When we can't sleep, we have this thought that we will never be able to sleep again. When that happens, Mum has to repeat the special sentences:

Lying in bed is just as good as sleeping.
If you needed sleep your body would put you to sleep.
And if you can't sleep, it's because you had enough sleep the night before.

Then the thought feels a bit better. We don't know why this works. We think it may be magic.

We went downstairs to ask for the special sentences. The door to the sitting room was ajar, and Mum and Dad were sitting on the red sofa with a bottle of wine, flicking through a brochure with pictures of smiling children. We stood there listening and never asked for the special sentences.

On weekends we and our younger sister Ella snuggle up under the covers of Mum and Dad's bed and watch the children's channels while they sleep more. It is always nice, as long as they are not upset with each other. Today feels a bit different. Firstly, because they called us to come up. Secondly, because they look

sad, but not like they have been arguing. We feel like they are
going to tell us something important. Ella, who is two, is making
her Sylvanian Families mouse jump up and down on the bedpost.
We tell her to stop playing, because it isn't that kind of day. Then
suddenly we know.

We know what has happened.

'It's Tom, isn't it?' we burst out. 'He's dead.'

Tom is our cousin. He was born with a hole in his heart. He
isn't even one yet.

'How did you . . . How did you know that . . .' Mum trails off.

She stares at us and has gone pale. She looks scared, and we're
not sure why. We smile, trying to make it okay again.

'Don't smile about this, okay, Lily? You don't smile about this.'

And that's when we know that we have done something very
bad.

'Yes,' Mum says. 'Tom died last night.'

Tom probably wasn't even dead before we said it.

We made it happen.

We know it.

Because we are bad.

On the last day of term, Mum takes us into the classroom. We
stop flat in our tracks, staring. Everyone is in fancy dress. We love
fancy dress. How had we not known?

'I didn't know it was a dressing-up day,' Mum says, looking
worried.

'Yes, for the last day of term!' says Miss Watts, beaming at us.
'Didn't you get the letter?'

4

New School

We have a fresh start. It's our first day at Buxton House. The manual says you must wear navy or red hair ties, and red ribbons if you like. We don't have any red ribbon, so Mum puts our hair in bunches and takes the red ribbons from our Lindt Easter chocolate bunnies. We wear a stripy blue-and-white dress, with a red cardigan, straw hat, white socks, and buckle shoes.

Things work differently at this school. At the old school, kids swarmed through the playground towards the building, slapping each other's backs, trading marbles and chatting. But here, you drive through large gates in your car and the headmistress stands by the door. You have to shake her hand and say 'Good morning, Mrs Woodson.'

Somehow, Mrs Woodson knows who we are. Perhaps it's because we are starting halfway through Year 3, so we're the only new girl. She asks a passing girl, Fiona, to take us to our classroom on the top floor. Fiona stares ahead and doesn't talk to us until we're about to go in. Then she links arms with us and hauls us in through the door, smiling: 'Good morning, Miss Hodge. Lily is the new girl in your class. Mrs Woodson has asked me to bring her to you. Lily, have a good day.'

Eleven heads turn to look at us, and we wonder why the class is so small. Perhaps the other children haven't arrived yet?

'Hello, Lily, nice to meet you. Everyone say 'Good morning, Lily.' Lily, put your hat in the box,' says Miss Hodge, pointing to a box full of boaters.

We take our hat off, and everyone starts laughing.

Scarlett, who has the next desk, whispers in our ear: 'It's the ribbons. In your hair. I know it says in the book of rules that you can wear them, but no one actually does.'

Our face burns redder than the stupid Lindt ribbons. We start to walk out of the class to rip them off, but Miss Hodge asks, 'Er, Lily, where do you think you are going?'

'Um. To the toilet?' Everyone laughs. A girl at the front says 'You have to ask if you want to go! And anyway, it's called a loo. Toilet is what common people say.'

Now they're in hysterics.

The noise is too loud for our head.

'Quiet down! Regardless of what you want to call it,' says Miss Hodge, her face softening, 'Maddie is right. You do have to ask for permission to leave the classroom if you want to go.'

She says we may go (so what was the point of that?). We find the loo, bin the ribbons, and scrape our hair into a ponytail. We repeat:

Fresh start.
Fresh start.
Fresh start.

We have sport at 11:30 am. As we're changing, trying to work out whether the B goes on the front or back of our gym shirts, Scarlett is hopping around, looking for a sock. 'I'm always the last one out!' She grins.

She can't tie her laces.

'Do you want me to help?' we ask. Scarlett looks pleased.

We squat down and try hard to focus. We also find laces difficult, but we want to get this right so she'll be our friend. Two minutes later, we're done. We stand up.

'Shall we go?'

Scarlett takes a step forward and tumbles. Oh, gosh; we've accidentally tied her laces together. Someone has been hurt, and it's our fault. We always knew we were a terrible person; now it has come true.

Scarlett is crouched in a ball, rocking and making weird noises. We bend down.

'Scarlett, are you okay? I'm so sorry. I didn't mean to.'

That's when we realise she is giggling hysterically.

'Hahaha! I can't believe you managed to tie my shoes together—you're just as bad as me!'

We have been at Buxton for a week now. Scarlett is our best friend. We do everything together and play imaginary animals at break time. We were wary of playing an imaginary game again, but it's going well. We are allowed three each. Scarlett has Rusty the red squirrel, an eagle called Gonzo, and Striko the horse, who has a lightning bolt on his forehead.

We made up Penelope the white squirrel, and Aslan the lion. I ask, 'Can I have a human as my third one?'

'Um . . . I'm not sure. Why would you want to have a human when you could have any really cool animal?'

'Because I already have a human, and I don't want her to be left out.'

'Oh, really?' Scarlett challenges. 'What is it called then?'

'She's a girl. And She doesn't have a name.'

'Well, you're obviously just making her up. Otherwise she would have a name.'

'Okay, She's called Victoria!'

'You just made that up!'

Scarlett looks cross. 'Okay, I'll ask Striko,' she says grumpily and turns to chat with a horse we can't see.

'Striko believes you have an imaginary human. But she can't come to the animal kingdom. Only animals can live there.'

'But humans are animals.'

'Well . . . Striko says only animal animals. Imaginary humans can't exist in the animal kingdom. Striko says if you want Victoria to live, you need to send her to the imaginary human kingdom, which isn't somewhere we play, so you won't see her again. But you get a third animal to replace her.'

'I'll take a cat as my third animal.'

The bad thing is that we are bottom of the class. We were never stupid before. Mum says it's not our fault. She says it's because classes here are smaller, so the kids get ahead, but if we work hard we can catch up.

We are in the bottom groups for everything, even English, and have extra lessons with Mrs Martin and Francesca and Holly. Today Mrs Martin tells us we do our Ks the wrong way.

'Lily, stop curling your Ks like that. That's the state school way. We do kicking Ks here.'

Francesca and Holly giggle, and we know they will tell the other kids, who already think we're common. Actually, they think lots of things. 'My mummy says your parents are too young,' Maddie had said yesterday.

'They said you were an 'accident.' Yuck!'

We are lying in our bunk bed, trying very hard to sleep because it is the first day of Year 4 tomorrow. Some things are okay. Mum has promised she will switch off the taps in the bathroom every night, so we don't have to worry about that.

But we still can't sleep. We sort of need the loo, but we don't want to go, because then we will have to turn the taps on, and that's too risky because Mum has gone to bed now, so she can't check that they are off. Every time we look at our watch, we feel even more worried, because morning is getting closer and we are still awake.

At about 11.15pm we heard our parents turn off the telly, put the chain on the door, and switch off the lights. We heard them pattering around upstairs for 10 minutes, and we thought about them brushing their teeth and putting their pyjamas on. But then that stopped too, and now the house is silent.

Everyone is asleep apart from us.

What if Ella stops breathing?

What if she is dying upstairs right now, gasping for her last breaths, and no one knows because they aren't there to hear? It's nearly midnight. Mum and Dad are definitely asleep.

If we don't check on Ella, who will?

Slowly we climb down our ladder, trying to tread like a mouse. Years of creeping round our room after bedtime have made us a pro. We know which floorboards creak and which don't, but it's still hard, because sometimes unexpected bits make noises. We tiptoe across from our bed to the door, which squeaks when it's opened.

If it only squeaks three times or less, tomorrow will be a good day.

Eeeeeeek, eeee, eeeee.

Our heart catches in our mouth.

We stand still for a minute. If Dad hears us, he will be cross and come and tell us off, because he has to work tomorrow.

The hallway and the stairs are better, because they're carpeted. We crawl up them—it's quieter that way.

Thankfully, Ella's door is open, because she is scared of the dark. We creep to the side of her bed. She is curled up on her side, her thick mop of brown curls covering her face. We brush them aside. We can hear her breathing, but to be sure, we hold our hand an inch from her mouth. We can feel her breath on our palm, so she must be alive.

We count nine of her breaths. Then we lower her duvet till it is just above her tummy. We place our hand on her chest. Her heart is beating. We count nine beats, but we're still not sure, so we count another nine beats, which takes us to 18. Leaving it like that would be bad luck—there have to be three sets—so we do another nine. Twenty-seven beats.

We think we must be done. It doesn't feel quite right, but if we stay here she might wake up. We pull up the duvet under her chin. We repeat the words:

Best sister ever.
Best sister ever.
Best sister ever.

We say it in our head three times so she doesn't wake up, but we focus hard on meaning it so she will be protected from bad things.

We make our way back to our room and check it's safe for us to go to sleep. We open our drawers, feeling around the insides with our hands. We worry that there might be someone, or something, hiding inside. We check our wardrobe and under the bunk bed.

The plug switches must be off so there isn't a fire in the night. We fumble around in the dark, checking they all point the right way. We creep up the ladder, and then we hang over the edge of the bunk bed to make sure there aren't any people lurking underneath in the shadows. We look:

Left, right.
Left, right.
Left, right.

Under the covers, we need to say the prayer. It is the last thing that has to be said before we can sleep. It is the best protection against everything going wrong. We have already done the prayer, but since then we left the room to check on Ella, so we need to start again:

Dear God,
Please protect our family.
Please do not let Ella die in her sleep.
Please do not let us wake up in the morning and our parents have left.
Please do not let the whole world turn to ice, so that we're the only ones who aren't frozen and we have to exist forever by ourselves.
Please make our parents happy and stop them not getting on.
Please make Scarlett always like us and be our best friend. Let the other girls in our class like us too and not think we're a bad person.
Please let this not be a game, let us not be the only person who really exists because everyone else is controlled by computers.
Please look after everyone in the world and make it better for the people who don't have homes, food, and water.
Please let us sleep now and remember that lying in bed is just as good as sleeping.

If our body needed sleep, it would put us to sleep.
And if we can't sleep tonight, it's probably because we had enough
sleep the night before.
Amen.

One round of the prayer takes a few minutes, and we repeat it twice to make three.

Often we get it wrong, and we have to do all three rounds again. Sometimes we don't get it wrong, but it sort of feels wrong. Then we have to start again too. That would make six rounds, so then we have to do another three to make nine. It's best to get all three rounds right first time.

The good thing is that this time we get all three rounds right on our first attempt. We lie back and shut our eyes tight. It must be time to sleep now.

But by now it's been about 30 minutes since we checked on Ella. How long does it take to die? Seconds. Imagine how many times she could have died by now. And there is no one to check on her but us. We'll go and see if she's still alive.

Just one more time.

5

Mum and Dad

We and Scarlett have just finished our swimming lesson. It is the worst part of the week, because the pool is freezing, and no matter what the teacher says, it's never okay once you're in.

Mum knows we hate the cold, so she is waiting with a towel for each of us at the changing-room door. The two of us wobble over, all plucked chicken skin and white webbed feet and hands, grabbing for the towels and chattering our teeth. Although we've started to feel that it's getting a bit babyish, the Disney print doesn't bother us right now. We wrap ourselves up in the soft faded blue of *101 Dalmations* having fun in a soapy bathtub; Scarlett has her own green towel from home.

Mum has got our stuff out of the locker; it's waiting for us in a pile on the low wooden bench that runs down the centre of the room. We dry our body, and then drop the towel on the floor and reach for our knickers.

'Don't drop your towel on the floor,' says Mum.

'Why?' we say.

'Because it's dirty.'

'But you're going to wash it when we get home.'

'Yes, but some things like floors are really dirty, and the washing machine doesn't get rid of all the germs.'

(This reminds us of something Dad said a few weeks ago: 'Always wash your hands when you get home after taking the Tube, because there's lots of invisible dirt on the poles from other people's hands; it's there even though you can't see it.')

'What if you wash it lots of times?' we ask. 'Does it go eventually?'

'Yes, probably eventually.' Mum's not paying attention anymore; she has turned to give Scarlett her socks. 'Sit on the bench when you put them on so you don't get your feet wet . . .'

Our towel is curled on the tiled floor. The lines between the tiles are filled with a spongy green slime we hadn't noticed before. Is this the super dirt Mum is talking about? No: Dad said it's invisible. We look at our hands, which are now less waterlogged and starting to look normal again. What about the lines on our palm? Are they filled with spongy green slime too tiny to see?

'How many times would you have to wash it to make it go away?'

'Oh . . . a few . . . Here, put your sweatshirt on.'

'Okay,' we say.

We resolve to wash our hands more often and more carefully.

Our special way of finishing our thoughts changes every few months. There's never a specific moment where the change is noticeable. At the moment, we tap each side of the chair we are sitting on three times. Then we triple it to make nine.

We smell our fingers one by one, carefully.

We look left, right, up, and down, three times.

We uncross and cross our legs three times and tap our feet up and down together three times.

Dad wishes we would stop.

He tells us he will get us a guinea pig if we promise to stop fidgeting so much, because it is unbearable to watch. We would like a guinea pig. We reason that we can move in a way that's less noticeable, or perhaps find another way to close our thoughts.

We make the deal with him.

Mum and Dad take Ella and us to a house outside London to get the guinea pig. We pull into the gravel drive of a large red-brick house. We open the car door to get out, and a little grey dog runs past. As we look at it, a thought pops into our head:

I hate that dog.

We clutch our head.

What a horrible thought, says my friend. *Why did you think that?*

I don't know, I say. *I love dogs. That dog looks friendly and nice.*

Ella is shrieking 'Where are the guinea pigs? I want to see the guinea pigs!' and the man and woman who come out the house give us a strange look.

'We don't have any—'

'They're in the basement!' interrupts Dad, winking.

Inside the house, there's a cage with lots of tiny fluffy grey puppies in it.

'We're getting a puppy!' says Dad.

We feel elated. A puppy! How amazing!

'Can we call him Tuffy?'

And then a pang. The older grey dog we saw on the drive must have been the mum. How can we take one of her children when I had such a horrible thought about her? And how will we look the puppy in the eye, knowing what I thought about his mum?

Our parents are rich now and have bought a wooden ski chalet in Chamonix in France. Everything about the chalet is great, and we are learning to ski, but the problem is, we have to drive to get there.

Mum and Dad have always argued, but it's getting worse. They argue about the most ridiculous things, and it's worse when we're in the car.

We don't want to take sides, but Dad is always shouting at Mum. According to him, everything she does is wrong. She doesn't want to fight, and cries, but it doesn't help, so she gets mad and shouts back. If he repeatedly runs his hands through his hair, you know he is really mad. Then you should keep quiet.

They are fighting before we even get to the end of our road.

By the time we get to France, they've argued about a million things. The main problem is that Dad has decided he doesn't like Mum's voice. He tells her it is high and piercing, and he hates it. Mum has put her Gucci sunglasses on. Since it's not sunny, she must be crying.

'And those huge glasses! Those fucking glasses!' screams Dad. 'They make you look fucking ridiculous!' He grabs them off her face and snaps them in half.

This is too much for Mum, who sat crying and not saying much through most of the last hour. She grabs a Scotch egg and smushes it in his face. She throws another at the windscreen. Dad swerves the car.

'Fuck!'

'STOP!' we scream. 'Dad, stop shouting at Mum. You're making her cry, and she hasn't done anything wrong.

'And Mum, put the Scotch eggs down.'

'You shut up, Lily!' says Dad. 'We are having an adult argument, and you bloody well stay out of it.'

In the car we used to calm ourselves down by doing our moving-around routines, but we promised Dad we would sit still. So now we either fidget very slowly so Dad won't notice, or we say our special sentences:

Everything is under control.
Their relationship is on the mend.
They love each other really.

Lately, we've found a better thing to do. We've realised Dad and Mum are probably bad, because otherwise he wouldn't treat her like that—and she wouldn't make him so unhappy. We don't want to end up bad like them, so we focus on counting up all the things we've done that day that could possibly be bad. We make a long list of them and think about whether what we did really was that bad.

Sometimes it turns out it wasn't bad, and we can excuse it.

Other times it was genuinely bad, and we have to think about it very hard to make sure we don't do it again. To be certain, we go through the list three times. Sometimes that goes wrong, and we have to go through it six more times to make nine. If that still goes wrong, we start again.

Of course, it's worrying that we've done bad things at all, but my friend reassures me:

The fact that you're thinking about it and trying to sort it out shows that you won't end up bad like them. The problem with them is that they don't care about it. You're going to grow up to be a good person, I know it.

It's so relieving to hear this—so thrilling and exciting to know that because She is here to help me, I have potential.

Knowing this makes their argument seem quieter, and though I'm still in the car, I'm not here really.

I'm in the future, 10 years from now, living in a stylish flat by the Thames and working in a very cool office with glass walls, a water cooler, and unlimited stationery. I don't have housemates, because I don't need them—I have my friend. And by this time we've worked it all out, and everyone loves us.

Thank you, I say, *thanks for everything.*

We're driving in the car through Chamonix. Mum and Dad are in the front, and we're in the back with Dad's sister, Auntie Sam. Dad is screaming at Mum about the fact that she doesn't even try to be good at skiing and he's sick of wasting money on her lessons. Mum is saying she does try. What happens next happens so quickly, we don't take it all in.

Mum unbuckles her seat belt, opens the passenger door, and jumps out of the car. We look to see where she will land. There is a patch of grass by the barrier, and she throws herself at it.

Her body curls in a ball, like a gymnast. Will she make it?

She has made it. She lands, bounces a few times, and rolls away from the impact. Then she is gone from view.

'Ian!' screams Auntie Sam. 'Ian!!!'

Dad keeps driving. Auntie Sam clutches our hand.

Please let her be okay.
Let her be okay.
Let her be okay.

Mum walks into the chalet hours later. We look her up and down. She looks okay. But what if she is hurting somewhere we can't see? We wrap our arms round her.

'Are you okay?'

Mum nods. She feels cold.

She has walked back.

She says everything will be fine between her and Dad. 'Sorry I did such a stupid thing.'

Then she buries her face in our hair, and our scalp starts to feel like it's raining.

At night, it doesn't matter what time we go to bed: our prayers and checks take hours before we can sleep. We share a bunk bed with Ella, and at first we wonder how we can do our checks with her there.

While we don't think there's anything wrong with checking things to be sure, we haven't seen anyone else do it and suspect it should be private.

By now, we've perfected the routine. We wait for Ella to be in the bottom bunk, and tell her we are going to the bathroom. Once there, we wash our hands three times, because otherwise we'll be kept up imagining all the things we can't see on our hands. We check the cupboard under the sink to make sure there is no one in it. We run our hand across the unsanded shelf, getting splinters in our palms. Then we check with our eyes:

Left, right.
Left, right.
Left, right.
Up, down.
Up, down.

Up, down.

We do the same on the bottom shelf.

We check the bath and sink taps, passing our hand under them nine times and saying:

They're off.
They're off.
They're off.

We take the loo roll out of the holder and check there is nothing underneath, three times.

Then we go back into our bedroom. We check behind the curtains three times, or nine if that doesn't feel right.

Ella always asks 'What are you dooooing?' and we always say 'I'm looking at the moon.' She asks why we couldn't see it the first time and we tell her to be quiet and go to sleep. Then we go over to her.

We feel that she is breathing in the special way and check her pulse.

It's harder to keep this secret. So we've decided to be half honest. We tell her we are just checking to see she is alive and well, like when you go to the doctor. In our head we repeat:

Best sister ever.
Best sister ever.
Best sister ever.

Then we get into our bunk. We check nine times that the duvet is tucked in so our toes don't get cold and wake us up, which would force us to start checking everything again. We check that our pillow is straight: the top must be a palm from the end of the bed and the sides a palm from the mattress edge.

Then we say the prayer and try to sleep. The problem is, having Ella close to us makes us feel even more like we need to check she is alive.

We creep down the ladder to check on her without waking her up. This must be the last thing we do before we get into bed, so we quickly check the bathroom and curtains again. Then we check Ella, before climbing back into bed and doing the duvet and pillow checks. Then we say the prayer again and try to sleep . . .

We check our watch. It's 5.00am.

We are.

So.

Tired.

We climb down again to check on Ella. We are checking her chest when she opens her eyes wide and sits bolt upright.

'Lily? Why do you keep doing this?'

'Shhh! Go back to sleep.' We stroke her head to calm her down.

'Lily,' whispers Ella, pulling the duvet up to her chin and looking at us with wide eyes.

'Am I dying?'

6

Swearing in Church

Every Thursday our whole school goes to the church down the road. It lasts 45 minutes, but it feels like hours. From the second we get into church until the second we leave, we can't stop saying rude words—in our head. Church is not the place for these words, but we can't make them go away.

Fucking boring-ass church. Crap, fuck, shit, wanker, cunt.

We look at the altar with the huge cross.

Fucking Jesus on a fucking cross. Crap, fuck, shit, wanker, cunt.

We sit down.

Fucking uncomfortable pew. Crap, fuck, shit, wanker, cunt.

The vicar starts talking about the love of Christ.

The vicar is a wanker cunt face. Crap, fuck, shit, wanker, cunt. Those robes just make him look like a massive dickhead.

We open our hymn books.

Fucking shit songs. Crap, fuck, shit, wanker, cunt.

What is *cunt*, anyway? *Crap* and *shit* mean poo, *fuck* is what adults do in bed. *Wanker* is someone who drives a car badly.

But what is *cunt*?

We are supposed to sing the hymns, but we are too scared the horrible words will come out instead and everyone will know how bad we are. Then the teacher tells us off and says we have to sing. We mouth the words.

Scarlett whispers in our ear, 'I don't believe in God.'

'Stop it,' we say.

'It's like believing in Father Christmas.'

'STOP IT!'

Why is Scarlett saying these things? Why won't she stop? Now we're definitely going to hell.

We sit on the steps during break, drinking our cartons of milk and watching the other girls skipping. We ask Scarlett why she doesn't believe in God.

Scarlett says when you're little, you get taught to believe in the Easter Bunny, the Tooth Fairy, Father Christmas, and God. When you turn 10, everyone says 'Okay, that stuff wasn't real, we just made it up. Except for God, he's real.' Scarlett says, 'If God existed, do you think the world would be so unfair? Do you think we would be sitting here enjoying our milk while kids die of thirst in Africa? And God would be just like: 'Well, it's their own fault. I did tell Eve not to eat that apple.' '

It's pretty funny; Scarlett is so smart.

'But I spend ages praying every night, and I constantly do all this stuff because I'm worried that if I don't, God won't protect me and my family.'

Now it's Scarlett's turn to laugh, though not in an unkind way. It's just a laugh that says *Why on earth would you do that?* 'Stop doing that,' she instructs. 'It's a waste of time. God doesn't exist.'

Thinking about it over the next few weeks, it seems Scarlett must be right; God does not exist. The prayer disappears, and the swear words in church start to seem more funny than scary. The funnier and less terrifying they are, the less often they come.

Finally, they stop coming at all.

When we get home today, Dad is on the sofa, staring into space. He fought with Mum yesterday, and we heard him say he was spending the night in a hotel because he couldn't bear to be in the house.

We wonder when he got back.

He doesn't hear us come in. He doesn't notice us when we stand in front of him.

We want to hug him and tell him everything will be okay, but he looks so sad.

We want to say *Thank you for working so hard, thank you for always looking out for us, thank you for being our dad. We understand that you only get angry because Mum doesn't make you happy, but you don't want to lose us.* But how can we say this?

Silently, we walk out of the room.

We are clever now. It took time, but we got there in the end. When we do exams, we are almost always in the top three. At the school prize-giving assembly, they announce who is top in the whole year and who is second and third. Usually Scarlett comes in top and we come in second. Then you get a book with a certificate in it to say well done. We like being smart. It's the only thing we've ever been any good at. We think that's why we get so upset when we don't understand something. It usually happens in maths. I tell myself it's fine, I'll get it the second time, but She starts saying:

Stupid.
Stupid.
Stupid.

She and I agree on almost everything, but very occasionally we have arguments. I don't think it's that bad to not get something the first time you are taught it. After all, you can't understand everything straightaway, and I'm still second top in maths after Scarlett.

But my friend says:

No, that's not how it works. If you don't get it, you're an
Idiot.
Idiot.
Idiot.

I try to focus on the words Mrs Johnston is saying and how I can apply them to the numbers in front of me. But She says it's much more important that we record that I have been stupid so we can go through it together later. I tell her that we won't have to record that I have been stupid if we learn it now.

But She says it's too late: not understanding the first time is as bad as never understanding. She tells me this so loudly that it cannot be disputed.

I try to compromise, and record in my head what I have done that is stupid while trying to understand Mrs Johnston.

It's an impossible task, and I know I'm going to cry. I feel it coming on; the tightness in my throat, the way the numbers start to go blurry. Then I see the tears splash on my textbook. I try to hide it, because I am 12: I am too old to be crying in class. I want it to stop, but the more I try not to cry, the more I do.

Mrs Johnston used to be nice about it. She used to give me a tissue and ask if I was okay, but lately she gets frustrated, and tells me I won't get away with this in big school. I know it must be annoying to have a kid in your class who bursts into tears all the time when you are trying to get on with your lesson, but it makes the tears come even faster, because between her and my friend, I feel like I must be a stupid baby.

I thought that once we had got rid of God, things might get better, but my friend has different ideas. She says,

There may be no God, but there are still things we need to protect ourselves from. And if we can't pray to God to make you an okay person who people like, we must make it happen ourselves.

School finishes at 5.20pm, and our au pair picks us up. Our au pair changes every year or so, because once she has learned English and qualified from the language school down the road, she gets a different job or returns home. At the moment, our au pair is called Illy and is from Slovakia. She is our favourite au pair ever. She is very tall, with short blonde spiky hair. She makes us laugh so much our tummy hurts and is always lovely to us. When Mum and Dad have fights or when we can't sleep, she lets us come into her room and watch TV.

When we get home, Illy gives us our dinner and we play a game, usually cards. Mum gets home from her office around 7.30pm. Dad gets back around 9.00.

Tonight, Mum gets back at 6.30, which is unusual. We are sitting playing cards in the living room when she says she wants to talk to us.

We panic. What have we done wrong?

We go into the kitchen with her. She sits down at the table and indicates for us to sit opposite her. She takes our hands in hers.

'Lily, are you okay?'

'Yes! Of course, Mum. Why?'

'Because I have a letter from school saying you keep crying in class and your teachers don't know why. School is asking if there's something going on at home that's upsetting you. Is there?'

'No! Not at all. Please don't worry. It's just I'm a bit of a baby when I don't understand something.'

'Okay. But I want you to know that if you ever were upset about something, you could tell me. Come here.' She pulls us into a hug. I should be safe and warm, but—

See?! She snarls. People have noticed that you're behaving weirdly. It's not all right to just sob your heart out over maths. Get it together!

We are about to graduate from Buxton House, which finishes at Year 8. Then it will be time to be mature. Everyone takes a 13-plus exam, but it's not necessary for Scarlett and us.

A few months ago, Scarlett told us that she had visited a boarding school in Kent with her parents, where they gave everyone personalised chocolate bars with 'Hambledon' written on the wrapping. Pupils could keep a goldfish in their dorm and there was a proper gym, swimming pool, tennis courts, great food—and it looked like Hogwarts!

We went to the school to do special tests. A couple of weeks later, we and Scarlett got letters saying we had passed. We are academic scholars and are expected always to be at the top of our class. Our name gets printed in big letters on a special wooden board in the entrance hall. It also means that while the other girls have to work hard for the next few weeks on the 13-plus, we get to bum around doing projects and making stuff, which is amazing.

What is also amazing is that Mum and Dad are getting divorced. They sat us down and told us last night. Ella cried, but we had to try hard not to shout with joy.

Dad will move out the house, and there will be no more fighting. This means we don't have to feel bad about leaving Ella behind when we go to Hambledon.

Before we leave Buxton, Mrs Woodson gathers the whole of Year 8 to have a talk. She stands at the front of our classroom, talking about protecting ourselves on the Internet.

She wants us to know that there are bad people out there, who might try to take advantage of the way we use websites. She is particularly concerned about Bebo, which is this new site where you connect with your friends and chat online. We all use it.

Mrs Woodson says she has taken a look at some of our profiles. She says that Athena's has a picture of herself in a bikini. Would Athena walk down the road to Clapham Junction in her underwear? No, she would not. Yet, Mrs Woodson tells her, what she has done online is exactly the same. She will speak to her privately afterwards.

Mrs Woodson says she is most concerned about bad people seeing our pictures and using them to masturbate, or finding our details and trying to track us down. She asks who in the class doesn't know what masturbation is. A few of us put up our hands.

'Right, er, okay,' she says, suddenly looking uncomfortable. 'It's when someone pleasures themselves by touching their private parts. They could do it by looking at photographs, or maybe touching another person to arouse themselves. Say, they could, er, touch your chest, or breasts, if you have them yet, or, er, even your bottom, to get pleasure. That would be called abuse.'

Mrs Woodson has gone red, but she takes a deep breath and carries on talking, as if the world isn't ending.

We are shaking in horror. Everything is going fuzzy, and we can't hear Mrs Woodson anymore.

All this time, when we were checking that Ella was alive and feeling her heartbeat, we have really been touching her chest over and over.

She asks: *Did you get pleasure from it?*

Only in the sense of being glad she was alive. Is that a bad sort of pleasure? Was it even pleasure? It felt more like relief. Either way, this is undoable. How could we not know we were abusing our own sister?

We mustn't check on Ella again: it is shatteringly clear that what we thought was saving her was really just the product of a dark impulse.

Thank god we are going to boarding school soon. Ella will be away from us. She will be safe. We will never, ever be able to hurt her again.

7

Most Apologetic Girl

School's out. Everyone in our year got into the secondary schools they wanted. To celebrate, Natasha has taken our class to stay at her country house in Norfolk.

We all hang out on the beach, taking turns to bury each other alive in the sand before paddling out into the waves. We get sunburned in that typically British way, having not bothered with the factor 50 Mum put in our backpack.

In the evening Natasha presents the Buxton House Leavers' Awards. We've already had the proper school prize-giving on the last day of term, where we won the English Cup, the French Plate, and the Science Shield.

This is different. We all sit in the garden, and Natasha hands out an award to each of us on a podium, while everyone cheers.

So far, Mia has won Prettiest Girl, Tabitha is Funniest Girl, and Scarlett is Cleverest Girl. Sarah battle-axes her way to Sportiest Girl, and Bryony looks suitably smug when she wins Best at Drama.

Then Natasha says our name, followed by our prize.

We walk up to her, trying to shake her hand while grinning so wide our cheeks hurt.

Everyone whoops. But really, it's not funny at all, because we have just won Most Apologetic Girl.

The only person who isn't laughing is Scarlett, and that tells us everything we need to know.

It's true: we have a tendency to apologise for our existence.

'Were you offended when I said that?'

'Said what?'

'I'm so sorry if it upset you when you got the wrong answer in history and I got it right. I didn't mean to make you look bad.'

'What question?'

'I'm sorry I was laughing when you walked past me in the corridor yesterday. I want you to know it was about something Mia said. I wasn't laughing at you.'

'You were laughing? I didn't notice.'

This time, things will be different.

This time, we won't turn up on the first day looking like an idiot. No ribbons.

This time, no one will think we're common.

This time, we won't apologise for everything.

There must be a way of dealing with worries that doesn't involve checking with everyone whether you have done something wrong. What could it be?

The question soon answers itself. Brushing our teeth at the sink next to Mia, we feel our elbow brush against her rib cage. We imagine a bruise forming under her T-shirt, spreading like spilled ink across her bones. We see it turning deeper shades of purple with every passing second, signalling internal bleeding and potential death.

Normally we would ask if she is hurt, and apologise for the damage inflicted. But in the past, people have responded strangely to this. They say things like 'You barely tapped me,' or 'When? I didn't feel anything.'

So we swallow the apology. It falls down our throat, landing in our stomach with a sickening bump. What next? We need to do something to make the sickness go, before it seeps into the rest of our organs and starts rotting them. We'll analyse it—work out if it really was bad. Just like we do when we're in the car. What we find out will tell us if we need to apologise.

We think it through and reason that we didn't touch her very hard at all. She didn't make any noise in response, and contact happens in confined spaces. These reasons make sense.

Every time we want to apologise, we remind ourselves of the reasons why we didn't do anything wrong, until finally, blissfully, unexpectedly, the fear that we've hurt her goes away. It feels like we are a magician who has waved his wand and vanished evil.

We apply this technique when Natasha's mum gives us cereal at breakfast and we say thank you, but she doesn't reply. We worry she may not have heard us and will think it impolite. But we don't say sorry and ask if she heard. Instead, we decide that she probably did hear, and even if she didn't, it's no big deal, because Bryony and Sarah didn't say thank you and no one is looking at them like the world is ending.

Breakfast finishes, and it's time to head to the beach. Scarlett and we have forgotten our sun cream, so we both dash upstairs to get it. The staircase is too narrow, and there isn't room for us both. We move in front of Scarlett. Instead of apologising for pushing past her, we think about it and reason that one of us had to reach the landing first, so we were simply being practical. Once back down, we don't apologise to everyone for stupidly forgetting our sun cream and for holding them up, because Scarlett also forgot hers. We know for a fact she isn't stupid, which means forgetting something can't be stupid.

Justifying why we don't have to apologise calms us down, but it doesn't quite make the need to apologise disappear, until we have repeated the reasons a few times.

So we decide that from now on we will go through reasons we don't have to apologise three times.

If that doesn't work, we will make it nine, and if that still doesn't work, we'll just keep saying them in multiples of three.

Right now, this sounds a little confusing, but we have the whole summer before we go to Hambledon.

We will spend it perfecting our technique.

We are 13. We're wearing a stripy green-and-pink Ralph Lauren polo shirt, skinny faded grey jeans, and gold pumps. Our hair is tied back in a messy bun.

Mum has helped us lug our trunk into our boardinghouse, Wimborne. Scarlett is here too, but she's in Aylingforde. That's fine—we didn't want to be in the same house anyway. We both agreed that if we were together all the time, we probably wouldn't talk to anyone else. We haven't seen her yet.

Mum, who has been feeling tearful since we saw the turrets of the red-brick castle on the hill, finally loses her cool. She's helping me put T-shirts in the drawer under my new bed when the waterworks start. Now she's wailing to everyone that she can't bear to lose her baby.

We are in a four dorm called Harper. Of our three new roommates, Ellie looks as if she's going to start laughing; Soo-jin blinks three times in quick succession. Alice, who has been at Hambledon since she was 11, is impossible to read.

We hiss: 'Mum, it's time to go.'

Our justification system—our way of not saying sorry all the time—starts to get out of control. Initially, the idea was to justify things we would normally apologise for, to make them go away without having to say sorry. But as we got better at it, we realised we could use the system to deal with pretty much anything.

Unless you can remember what went wrong, though, you cannot put it right. So we take the first letter of each worry and put it in a list. We continuously repeat the list in our head until we have a quiet moment to go through them all.

If we find a way of justifying the action, it becomes a green word. When we can't justify it, it is marked as a red word. We must remember and learn from it so we don't do it again.

Green words stick around for a day, being reevaluated to check that they definitely weren't that bad, and then get left behind at some point between when we fall asleep and when we wake up the next morning.

Red ones can continue to be carried forward for several days until we find a way to excuse them.

If we've done something really bad, we have to accept that there is no way of excusing it. Then it becomes a very red word, and we see its letters spelled out bolder in our head, flashing an angrier crimson colour. It then goes into the Master Archive, which is the area in our head where we store all the really bad things we've done. We visit those words about once a week, to see if anything about them has changed.

Our list from today is **EHHCSBR**:

ENTER: When we came through Wimborne's main doors, Mum and we were holding our trunk, and we brushed past another girl. Will that girl think we were being a pervert, trying to touch her?

HANDS: Was my hand sweaty when we shook my new housemistress's hand in the entrance hall? If so, will she think I'm disgusting?

HELLO: When we met Alice, we said 'hello' and she replied with 'hey.' Is hello the wrong way to introduce yourself? Will she think we are weird?

CRYING: Does everyone think we're a ridiculous baby because Mum cried?

SHIRT: Mum dried her eye on her shirt. Will they think we're disgusting and have been brought up to clean facial leakages using items of clothing?

BUM: After Mum left, we were talking to Alice about her favourite bands and she turned round to get something out of the drawer under her bed, but she did it so quickly we couldn't look away, and our eyes skimmed her bum for a second. If she saw, will she think we're a pervert?

RUMBLE: Our stomach rumbled when we were all sitting in the room talking. Did anyone hear, and if so, do they think we are vile because our body made a disgusting noise?

EHHCSBR.
EHHCSBR.
EHHCSBR.

We sit on our bed and try to quickly sort our head. We anticipate this could take a few minutes. Luckily, Alice, Ellie, and Soo-jin are also sitting on their beds, having a conversation about Ellie's old school.

With the right amount of nodding and smiling in (hopefully) the right places, we'll be able to look like we are involved in the conversation while sorting through **EHHCSBR**.

Before we repeat the words, we must do the movements. Years ago, when we promised Dad we would stop fidgeting in exchange for a pet, we learned to be subtle with them. Now, we keep them as imperceptible as possible by only making tiny moves. We are grateful to him for this; we wouldn't want to be marked out by some noticeable physical quirk.

We tap our feet on the floor nine times, invert our feet to the left and right, pull our sleeves down on each side, and tuck our hair behind our ears.

We repeat:

Tap, invert, sleeves, hair.
Tap, invert, sleeves, hair.
Tap, invert, sleeves, hair.

Sleeves is a reminder for us to pull our top down as far as possible to cover our hands; they are always rosy as clown cheeks from washing them too much. 'It looks like you're wearing red gloves,' Ella said previously, 'or like you dipped them in a cauldron of boiling water.'

It is best to keep them hidden.

Invert. A couple of years ago, we sprained our ankle and it never got completely better, so sometimes it gives out. When that happens, our foot falls in on itself and we look like a freak who can't even walk. *Invert* had been a red item for so long, we gave it special status. Why do we make ourselves repeat an embarrassing action? No idea.

Where do *tap* and *hair* come from? No idea either.

After the moving actions, we repeat all the words on the list three times. It must be done quickly and rhythmically, as if reading aloud from a shopping list. If the rhythm between the words feels wrong, or if there is a word that can't be recalled instantly, the whole thing must be done again.

ENTER, HANDS, HELLO, CRYING, SHIRT, BUM, RUMBLE.

ENTER, HANDS, HELLO, CRYING, SHIRT, BUM, RUMBLE.

ENTER, HANDS, HELLO, CRYING, SHIRT, BUM, RUMBLE.

Then we assess the words individually:

ENTER: Brushing past that girl was clearly an accident. She probably didn't even notice. And anyway, it could have been her who brushed past us.

HANDS: We have felt our hand against our face nine times since to check and can confirm that it is dry and there is no need to worry about the handshake.

HELLO: Clearly saying hello is wrong and uncool. This must be remembered.

CRYING: Mum cried, and it was ridiculous. There is no

getting around the fact that everyone probably thinks we're a mummy's girl.

SHIRT: They probably didn't notice Mum wiping her face on her shirt. Since we don't ever do this ourselves, we can prove over time that we are not disgusting.

BUM: Alice was facing away from me, so she could not have noticed the bum glance. The others were talking, so probably didn't notice either.

RUMBLE: Everyone's stomach rumbles sometimes, and it is very unlikely they heard it, as everyone was talking loudly.

In our head, we colour the actions according to what is now okay and what is still bad. **H**ELLO and **C**RYING are still red, so must be carried over to a new day.

Before the routine can be closed, we must repeat our three mottoes:

In the end it is all done.
Anger only hurts the one who feels it.
If you want nice friends, you must be nice to them.

These mottoes get us through the day. The first reassures us that at some point we will have learned enough from our routines to not do them again. Two and three are equally important, because without them we'd express unacceptable feelings like annoyance and anger. We fear that we could become nasty and violent. Finally we do:

Tap, invert, sleeves, hair.
Tap, invert, sleeves, hair.
Tap, invert, sleeves, hair.

Then we land in Blank Slate, which is the time where we have come as close as possible to our head being clean—before we do another bad action. Blank Slate can last anything from 10 seconds to a few minutes. Unfortunately not much of the day is spent in Blank Slate, but when we are there, it's a euphoric place: a gift, an unrivalled vantage point, from which everything seems crisper and better defined. Arriving in Blank Slate feels like resurfacing after being under the sea—that first breath you take when your lungs are greedy for oxygen and the joy of sun and sky hits you all at once. She is always kind to me when we get there.

All is well now, She soothes.

We float on our back in sparkling turquoise waters, a silky ocean current threading over our body, between our fingers. Relief pulses through our veins, as we kick back to shore.

8

Hambledon

On the weekends all the girls in the same year in our boardinghouse loaf around in the common room, watching endless DVDs, documentaries, and reruns of *Hollyoaks*.

We make 'the boat,' where we push the two sofas together to form a square, and then dump all the comfy cushions in the middle. There's a door to the kitchen, and everyone takes it in turns to do the 'toast run' so that we have TV snacks. We try to avoid our turn, for we see the invisible dirt on our fingertips seeping angrily into the spongy white slices of loaf: E. coli, salmonella, listeria. At the beginning of term we made toast for everyone, and Ellie got sick the day after. Enough said.

A collective popcorn is made about once a day. We try to get out of the kitchen when the microwave is on, because Mum once said you shouldn't stand near one in case the rays escape and fry your organs. Most girls in our year have already got their period, and we can't help wondering if the reason we haven't had ours is because we fried our ovaries in the past. Mum wouldn't have a microwave, just to be on the safe side, but Grandma had one, so it's possible the radiation occurred when we were younger.

Either way, there's no point compounding the damage.

There's normally a power struggle about what we watch. Alice likes gruesome horror stories and films about planes going down with people clutching their babies and shrieking, but she'll settle for a documentary about serial killers. Ellie would rather watch Disney classics. The rest of us slot somewhere in between. Personally, we like the serial killer shows, because it's a relief to know there are people out there worse than us.

Recording our mistakes has become our full-time occupation. Most words are generated when interacting with other people, like at mealtimes or when everyone is hanging out in the dorm. At these busy times, remembering everything that has been done wrong is such an effort that there's no time to actually work through the list. In quieter moments, like being in assembly, doing homework, or pretending to read a book, we get a chance to stop and review the day's data so far. It's called a Pause. By rights then, watching TV should be bliss. Not much talking gets done, and there's ample time to go over everything. Yet nothing about these routines is pleasant. It's like making yourself answer the same maths question over and over and coming up with a different answer every time, even though you don't actually like maths, so there's no conceivable reason why you would want to occupy all your free time with it.

She tells me that over time doing these lists will make us perfect, but it's little consolation. Every day feels like an unrelenting slog of words generated, letters compiled, actions reviewed—with nothing to show for it but exhaustion and despair.

At 7.00am every weekday, the Wimborne alarm screeches throughout the house. We roll over, not wanting to open our eyes, because within five minutes letters will be dancing and cartwheeling across our brain.

We swing our legs out so they dangle over our bed, reaching down to our top drawer to pull out some pants before grabbing our school uniform from the chair. Actions start to be recorded:

STARE: *As we got up to sit on the side of the bed, our eyes made contact with Soo-jin. She was sitting on the end of her bed in a bra. Will she be disgusted and tell everyone Lily is a pervert?*

UNDER THE DUVET: *The others get ready quite openly, but we prefer to take our pyjamas off and dress under the duvet so no one sees our body. As we pulled our pants up, we made a funny grabbing motion with our hands by accident. What if someone thinks we were masturbating?*

REACH UP TO GET BOOK: *We got off the bed and reached up to get our maths textbook from the top shelf. It felt like our skirt might have lifted up a bit at the back. What if everyone thought we were flashing them because we derive pleasure from exposing ourselves?*

MATHS HOMEWORK: *Soo-jin asked if we'd done the homework. We were a bit sleepy and said 'Which homework?' This was idiotic because maths is the only lesson we have together.*

School uniform on, we brush our teeth with Alice.

BREATH: *Alice said 'Come and brush your teeth with me,' so we both walked along the corridor to the cubicles. She asked us a question and we turned to her to reply. What if our breath stank because we hadn't brushed our teeth yet?*

DREAM: *Alice told us she dreamed last night about a train going round her head and knocking people dead. She looked at us expectantly. We don't think we expressed as much concern and sympathy as she expected.*

MIRROR: *Alice came and shared our cubicle. We accidentally looked in the mirror, which we must avoid doing in front of other people. Will she think we are vain?*

The alarm sounds again at 7.15am. and the whole of Wimborne files downstairs to the common room for roll call. A range of offenses are committed.

SQUEAL: *Mrs Grove called our name. We meant to say 'Yes' normally, but it came out squeaky, and everyone is going to think we have a horrible stupid voice.*

EYE CONTACT: *We caught the eye of a Wimborne first-year by accident. Will she think we were trying to groom her?*

The others can be summarised as follows:

WHISPER
MUDDY
ELBOW
SMILE
JUICE DISPENSER
CROISSANT SPILL
ATE SLOWLY
THANK YOU
THREE

BRUSHED LEGS
SAT WITH NAOMI

Once we're in assembly, it takes about 10 minutes for the hall to be full. The chaplain marches onto stage to tell us that Jesus has come to save us, generating the first Pause of the day. It's time to address the list so far.

We go through it three times:

SURMBDMSEWMESJCATTBS.
SURMBDMSEWMESJCATTBS.
SURMBDMSEWMESJCATTBS.

A few more letters pop up while the chaplain talks, and we slot them in at the end.

Between three and 10 letters are normally generated on the way to class. While you don't communicate in class as much as in everyday life, interaction is still required. When the teacher is talking, you can pretend to listen while actually reviewing words, but you might not finish if you're interrupted by something inconvenient like a worksheet. So classes are Half Pauses.

Full Pauses include going to the toilet, having a shower, and, most importantly, the time before we go to sleep. Full Pauses are used to review all words created that day, though the depth of the review can be tailored to the time available. A toilet review must be quick (otherwise someone might think we've gone for a huge shit, and that would generate so many letters it doesn't bear thinking about). We get longer in the shower, say 20 minutes, but we can only focus on reviewing once we have washed our full body three times, or nine if we still don't feel clean. We go over the list until someone bangs on the door and shouts to hurry up. Bedtime has an indefinite time allocation.

At the end of the day, there tend to be between 100 and 350 letters.

The day's list must be analysed before we sleep, along with the red letters carried forward from previous days. We lie on our bed re-sorting the letters into red and green afresh, deciding what is definitely green and can be discarded, and what is so serious it must be taken with us into tomorrow. This takes up to four hours.

A Christmas tree materialises in the Wimborne entrance hall, and our housemistress is sitting next to it, tapping away on her BlackBerry. When she looks up, she sees Georgia and ourselves bashing the snow off our shoes on the doormat outside.

'Hey, you're first back,' she calls. 'You guys get to decorate. I've got to go do some jobs.' She kicks a cardboard box of baubles and tinsel in our direction and disappears down the corridor.

We couldn't be happier to oblige. We untangle the lights and wind them round a few times, before starting on the plastic red and gold baubles. It takes about 20 minutes. Finally, Georgia lifts us on her shoulders and we plonk the star on top.

Alice arrives back from maths, pulls the rest of the tinsel out the box, and takes it upstairs to Harper. We follow.

At her heels like a dog, She sneers. *It's pathetic.*

We add **C**LINGY to the list. Up in Harper, Ellie and Soo-jin have hung fairy lights from the curtains. The four of us sit on the floor in the middle of our twinkly grotto, cutting scrap paper into snowflakes. 'I Kissed a Girl' blasts from the speakers on repeat.

They are bitching about teachers. It takes me a moment to

realise they're looking at me. 'Well?' probes Ellie. 'Don't you have a teacher you don't like?'

We've been cutting quietly while revising a list, but verbal interaction is now required. This means we'll have to start all over again on this list after we've spoken, which is annoying and panic-making. Frustration prickles across our skin like static. But at the same time, it's nice to know there are people nearby who stop you fading away altogether.

Because here's my friend's worst thing about being in a dorm: our lists get interrupted. And my best: our lists get interrupted.

One biology lesson a few months later, when the sun is shining brightly through the windows behind the whiteboard, and Georgia is sitting next to us drawing patterns with her protractor on her worksheet, we learn the shocking truth.

We are a boy.

We can't believe we didn't realise before.

We find out when Mrs Nelson says we don't look like we are concentrating very hard and tells us to read aloud from the textbook to the class. We were two letters away from finishing a routine that had been going on since we sat down at the beginning of the lesson. We want to scream. We want to throw the book at her and tell her she has cost us half an hour of our life that we will never get back. We don't, because anger only hurts the one who feels it. Instead, we sit up straight, smooth down the page, and read aloud carefully:

Jan was looking at her chromosomes under a microscope in biology class, when she saw something unusual. Instead of having XX chromosomes like a normal girl, she had XY. Shocked and confused, Jan went to the doctor, who explained that due to a genetic mutation, she had been left with an XY genotype, which explains why despite being 16, Jan has never had a period.

Although Jan had lived all her life thinking she was like other girls because she was born with a vagina, she has no ovaries. Instead, she has internal male testes. While Jan will not be able to have children, she has recently started dating Tom. Tom understands about her condition and is supportive. Medication means Jan can expect to live a relatively normal life.

And that's when we know. We are like Jan. It explains everything. All that time spent worrying that we didn't get our period because what happened when we were younger damaged us and made us infertile, we were focusing on the wrong thing. We don't even have any ovaries. It's clear that we are a hermaphrodite. It explains why we have so much hair on our arms and legs, and why we have no boobs or bum and the body of a boy.

We clamp down hard on our lip so the scream doesn't escape, because no one is ever going to want to marry a boy who thinks like a girl.

9

Running from Words

After biology, Georgia and us dump our files and books at Wimborne, change into our sports kit, and head to Upper Ock.

Upper Ock is a giant sports field on the grounds, but it's so far away from the main buildings (you have to walk through the rose garden to get there) it feels like somewhere else altogether. Every day after school for hours the two of us run round the 400-metre track, which is painted white on the grass.

Georgia does this because she is tipped to run for Great Britain in the 2012 Olympics. I do it because running is the antidote.

I align my body with the start line and fill myself with breath.

Georgia executes all sorts of warm-up drills, because her coach says you can't train properly without doing them. She has tried to persuade me to do them with her.

Georgia does not understand that I am not training.

She lives in the future—hears 'running' and 'gold medals' in the same sentence, pictures herself jogging victory laps around stadiums and ascending podiums, probably to her favourite music. This is her goal, and she is running towards it.

My goal is much less heroic and exists purely in the present. In fact, I'm not sure it even counts as a goal. I am not trying to achieve a personal best; I am trying to outrun my friend.

Being less fit would actually make it easier.

When I started running with Georgia a few months back, my pulse would roar in my temples; hotness would rise to my hairline; the cold air would coat my lungs with a bloody metallic tang. The physical discomfort alone made it pretty much impossible to focus on any lists. But the better I get at running, the less quickly I achieve my goal, because now it takes much longer to get to the level of physical pain needed to reach distraction. At first I set myself three laps an evening, and that would be enough to switch my head off.

As I became tolerant, I upped it to six, nine, 15 . . .

18, 21, 24. . .

Now I'm on 42, which is approximately 10 miles. Georgia tells me I will injure myself. She does not understand that I do not care.

One, two, three—my body tenses, I push up from my back foot and hurl myself into forward momentum along the track.

My friend whispers:

TCNDUCTOSCLSKEAYJLPRD.

Not now, I say.

She says:

TCNDUCTOSCLSKEAYJLPRD.

I focus hard on my lane, studying the blades of grass that stand coated in stiff white paint, making me think of 100,000 mini plaster-of-paris casts.

A 100,000? That can't be right. It must be more than that. Each painted line is probably 10 centimetres thick and definitely 400 metres long. There are eight lanes requiring a total of nine painted lines to make the track. So all I need to do is count the number of blades of grass in a 10-by-1-centimetre area of one of the lanes and multiply it by 40,000 and then multiply that by nine, and then I'll know how many mini plaster casts there really are—

TCNDUCTOSCLSKEAYJLPRD.

Her voice is insisting, wheedling, difficult to unhear. It will only be deafened by a high-intensity pain in my body, so I up the pace. The cows in the neighbouring field chomp disinterestedly on grass and gaze over the fence. The concept of running laps must be bizarre to a cow, mustn't it? Cows! That's another one, that's easier than grass, how many cows are there in the field? One, two, three, four—must run faster, go, go, go!—five, six, seven, eight—

TCNDUCTOSCLSKEAYJLPRD!!!

She shrieked that one — She's a banshee; She's a spoiled child demanding the whole of me, tugging at my shorts as I try to run past her, and . . . oh! I'm going to give in again.

She isn't going to be distracted by grass or cows.

Fine, fine, I say, and start to go through the letters with her. She's leading the routine, shuffling letters efficiently into red and green like piles of cards, saying when things are okay, chastising when they are not and sending me to the scarlet kingdom. We're on **U**—

Did I appear noticeably **U**PSET in biology after reading the passage out loud? Did anyone notice and guess our secret?

—when I try to trick her.

In the part of my brain closest to her, I appear to be happily going through the motions of letters **C**, **T**, and **O**, but closer to my forehead, in the space I am sometimes able to keep her out of, I make the decision to keep going faster every 30 seconds. It's a subtle increase, so slight She won't notice it, hopefully, until it's too late. I keep my breath even and press on for the next few laps.

As I pass her, Georgia calls out, 'You're flying round!'

My friend realises she's being gradually muted and lets out a shout of anguish.

But it's too late for her.

She'll pay me back later, but this is my time now. 'I know!' I grin. I steel my gaze ahead and accelerate. Some sort of toxicity is seeping into the muscles in my legs. We learned— in biology—that this is lactic acid, which builds up during anaerobic respiration when you can't get enough oxygen to the body parts that need it. It's perceived to be a bad thing, but I use it like rocket fuel.

The remaining letters rush out my ears, shimmying down underneath my vest top and shorts, landing in my socks before tumbling out and unraveling in ribbons behind my shoes. I imagine—and I know this is bad—my friend out of my head and onto the track in front of me, and me running her down like a car. The force of something else that can, when you think about it, really only be me, clasps my rib cage and begins squeezing the bones inward—I'll run out of air soon, well good, do your worst and—

The rush. The rush of this open field where I can see for miles: the other fields beyond the fence that turn into unkempt meadows, and the woods that get smaller and smaller, the winding toy gardens taken from the grounds of a princess's doll's house. The rush of knowing that whoever owns this field will never know it like I do, which means that in the world after time, where money doesn't matter and no one cares for territorial battles, it will all belong to me.

Georgia appears by my side, challenging me to a lap race. I don't know why I agree. I always lose. I suppose it's because I know she needs the rush of beating someone like I need the rush of escaping the letters. We're matching each other's speed for the first 200 metres, and I anticipate the moment where she will overtake me like she always does. It doesn't seem to come. At 300 metres I realise I'm a couple of strides ahead of her, and then there's nothing but me against the wind, each footfall sending me bounding forward on higher and higher springs, carrying me across the finish line, swiftly followed by Georgia a few seconds later.

She is doubled over, her hands on her knees, her badly dyed blonde hair, which is now ginger, swinging like vines against the tips of the green and white blades of grass. 'I couldn't keep up with you!' she puffs.

'I'm sorry,' I say instinctively.

'What on earth do you have to be sorry for?' She laughs, patting me on the back.

They should bury me here, the place where I run until my heart beats apart from all other noises, isolated like a drum removed from a score of hateful music I never wanted to play.

10

Stumbling

6.30pm. Canteen. We witness the disorder parade: anorexics pushing their food around with redundant forks, taking a still-full tray up to the counter when the matron looks away; socially anxious girls sitting alone at a table for 30 or looking self-conscious behind a DIY fringe; a morbidly obese girl having double doors opened for her, sweating under the buffet lights—getting upset when told she can't have seconds.

We sit with our friends. They are talking about Zac Efron and Vanessa Hudgens, their voices refracting off plates, glasses, and tables; booming surround sound. We imagine ourselves covered in egg cartons, like the bedroom of a rock star before he is a rock star, with holes cut for our nose. If the voices were muffled, would they be more bearable?

It doesn't help that we can't eat—can't look at our plate without imagining all the food it has ever had on it: a swarm of mashed potato, vinaigrette, bolognaise, gravy, and macaroni cheese. Six hundred people eat in this room three times a day. It is inconceivable that our plate has not previously been used by someone with poor personal hygiene.

How reliable is the school dishwasher?

How many people have sucked on this spoon?

Had those people ever given a blowjob? If so, when, and did they brush their teeth in the morning?

The plate teems with wet pork, beans, and saliva.

We shake our head. It's just a plate.

Shiny, white, sparsely covered.
Shiny, white, sparsely covered.
Shiny, white, sparsely—

No use. It is dirty, lethal, overused. Somehow we are standing up and gripping our tray. 'Everything okay?' Georgia asks, her face a map of concern. We nod dumbly and run to the used tray counter. The smell of half-eaten food and used spit makes us gag. We try not to breathe, but the queue of girls handing in their trays to the women on the other side is too long, and inside we're jumping up and down. We'll need air soon.

We're at the counter with our tray. A woman is on the other side, wearing an apron and blue latex gloves, scraping food juices into the bin. Her gloves are covered in it—beetroot, chicken, ketchup, mayonnaise up her arms.

She looks like she has just delivered a child.

A crash. Smashing glass, clattering cutlery. Our tray is on the floor, our hands splayed like starfish. We are momentarily frozen. Silence, heads turning, then clapping; the standard boarding school response. We should laugh it off, get a mop, a dustpan and brush, anything—too late.

We are running from the canteen, double doors swinging behind us as we head out into the night.

We're happy when half term rolls around. We are spending the week at home, and Ella, who has survived two and a half years without us checking up on her, is grinning on the doorstep when we pull up in the car with Mum.

The three of us shuffle though to the kitchen and catch up over big mugs of sweet tea. Ella fills us in on events of the term—her main part in the upcoming school play; the new friendship group she has fallen in with; the geography teacher she doesn't like. On the whole, then, things are going as well as they could be.

That is, until we meet with the thought that changes everything. Uninvited and entirely dark, it arrives on the back of some very bad news. When Ella goes upstairs to learn her lines, Mum tells us her best friend Gemma has cancer, and that the doctors have said it is probably terminal.

This is what we say out loud: 'Oh, no. That's awful. I'm so sorry, Mum. You must be really sad. . . . But Gemma is so full of life. She's got more energy and fight in her than anyone I know. If anyone can make it, it's her.'

But in our head this is what is said:

I want Gemma to die.

This thought stops our world, makes us shake, demands we acknowledge that nothing will be the same again.

I want Gemma to die.
I want Gemma to die.

'Are you okay, darling?' asks Mum. 'I know, I know. It's awful. I feel the same.'

I want Gemma to die.

The thought bounces from one corner of our brain to the other, like a teenage miscreant who is too old to be on a bouncy castle but who won't get off. The thought that this is wrong is like the castle's furious owner forced to clamber onto it to remove the adolescent, stumbling and swearing. The delinquent squeals: 'Catch me if you can, old fucker, catch me if you can!'

It would be comical if it wasn't horrific.

Why is this happening? I ask my friend. *And why is it my thought and not our thought? How did you get off so easily?*

She replies: *I don't know.*

What can I do? I ask.

She shrugs. *I never knew you were this bad*, She replies, sounding at a loss.

More than anything, we want to ask Mum why this is happening, but we can't. She loves Gemma. She'll think we're a murderer, and then she'll remember what happened with cousin Tom. How could she live with herself, knowing her child was so evil?

She couldn't.

A few days later, Gemma comes over to see Mum for a cup of tea.

Normally we like seeing Gemma, but this is torture.

The bad thought has been booming around our head,

swelling to an indefinite magnitude. We've accidentally added it to certain things like pens, radiators, and trainers, so that every time we see those, the thought instantly returns. We've hidden all our pens and our trainers so that they won't trigger the thought—but we can't pull the radiators off the walls. We try to think of anything else, but it doesn't work.

I want her to die.
I want her to die.

We make an excuse and leave the room, running up the stairs two at a time to our bathroom. We curl up in a ball and rock back and forward. Normally the cold tiles make us feel better, but today they don't.

We hear Mum asking Gemma how she's holding up. Their voices drift up the staircase.

Those are the voices of honest, good-hearted people. They are the voices of people who are fundamentally different from us.

11

Special Needs Department

Somewhere along the way, GCSE exams rear their ugly heads, and we can't complete them in the allocated time. The letters pop up and have to be addressed before we can even think about working out how many cakes Ahmed and Brian will have left at a bake sale if they have 243 of them and sell 23 percent within the first hour. When we do the practice papers, we get about a third of the way through by the time everyone else has finished.

If we don't complete the papers, we will most likely fail and have our scholarship taken away. We've heard about something called Extra Time. It gets given to people with learning difficulties. If you go to the Special Needs Department, you can be assessed to see if you qualify.

We sign up for an assessment. Two weeks later a plump woman in a baby-blue suit with short crimped brown hair comes to the department to test us. She goes through sheets of tests with us, licking her finger to turn the pages in that disgusting way of older people.

She asks us endless questions about circles, puzzles, and patterns, recording the time we take to answer them. We answer all her questions as slowly as possible. After an hour, she disappears to a little room to assess her notes. We wait at

the desk, trying to make all the lies we have told to get to this
stage not be so red.

*We had to do it because we'd be letting down the school and our parents
if we fail our exams.*

*We had to do it because if we failed our exams, everyone would think
we were stupid.*

*We had to do it because the lists are the focus of our existence, and
this is the only way they can be protected and we can still do our exams.*

Blue-suit woman comes back, patting our arm and smiling like
she's about to tell us we are dying from some incurable disease.

No one else will suffer if we get Extra Time. This is a safe untruth.

She informs us that we are 'a slow processor.' We will be
given the full amount of Extra Time and extra classes to help.
Sympathy drips from her words like honey. She understands
that we are academically very strong, but these problems will
hold us back if they aren't addressed. We smile and try to look
reassured by her promises that we now have everything we need
to succeed, and that it was brave of us to ask for help.

Over the next few weeks, we start weekly classes in the Special
Needs Department. Mrs Hall, the teacher, is plump and looks
like a mole. She is kind to her core. We think she sees through
the slow-processor diagnosis, because instead of focusing on
'improving our reasoning skills' as instructed, after two sessions
she asks us about our files and our work notes. We admit to her
that we don't file anything or write many notes in class.

She asks us if it's because we are thinking about something
else. We don't have the heart to lie to her, even if it means the

time is taken away. We say yes, it's because we are thinking about other things. Thankfully she doesn't ask what. She tells us to bring a file from a different subject each week.

Mrs Hall brings us in a box of Celebrations every week. She pours them out across the desk and tells us to eat as many as we like, because she says we need fattening up. The two of us guzzle our way through the box, and she chats about her son Michael and her three dogs.

We sort through the notes we have managed to write, and the hundreds of worksheets and handouts that have ended up piled under the bed in our dorm because we don't have time to organise them. The papers sift through her podgy hands and into appropriate plastic folders and topic sections in a whir of efficiency. Something about her puts us at ease. By the end of term, everything is beautifully highlighted, subheaded, and in its place. If anyone checked, there would be nothing to indicate that we weren't the perfect student.

The morning of GCSE chemistry is a letter avalanche. On stressful days, more things are done wrong and must be recorded. I wonder whether we generate letters simply because we're more anxious and not because recording them serves any inherent purpose. She shrieks:

NO! NO!
That idea is ludicrous. The correlation is false: the words are valuable in and of themselves and caused by real mistakes and nothing else.

I've never seen her get scared before, but something about my suggestion made her tremble. I saw a vulnerability I didn't know existed. Why?

Today, Wimborne is united. We have an early breakfast and sit in silence, forlornly spooning cereal into our mouths. Textbooks are spread across the table, and between mouthfuls, everyone is trying to absorb as much as possible about ionic bonding.

What is going through their heads is unknown, though Ellie is weeping. For our part, we have 74 letters to account for. It's 8.10am, and the exam begins at 9.00. No time for last-minute revision. We frantically try to go through our list without doing anything else wrong.

We walk across to the sports hall at 8.45am. Alice tells everyone who is going on about how badly they are going to fail to shut the fuck up, since we all know the only person who is going to fail is her.

The doors to the hall open at 8.55. The whole year files in, and hundreds of shoes squeak across the floor and chairs squeal as they are pulled out from under desks. 'You'll do great,' Mum texted this morning. 'You've done so much work. You deserve to nail it!'

What really happened was that over the Easter holidays, we sat upstairs in our bedroom at our desk in front of the window, with textbooks and notepads spread out in front of us, for about 10 hours a day. Mum brought us snacks on little saucers and kept showing up with mugs of tea. We used this time as an extended Pause. We went over all the bad things we'd done since we started Hambledon, focusing hard on the things that were so red they'd made it into the Master Archive. This was mixed in with assessing the minutiae of day-to-day things that made it onto our list during the holidays.

All in all, the revision we actually did was limited.

It's 8.56 when we find our desk. By focusing hard and engaging in as little pre-exam chat as possible, we've managed to assess 56 of the now 102 letters. If we're going to start the exam on time, four minutes remain to deal with the rest.

We're stuck on 57. There is no way to excuse it.

VAIN: We were waiting with Naomi and Trish to meet the rest of the house for breakfast. We were focusing hard on going through the words when Trish said 'Stop staring at yourself in the mirror, you gimp.' We realised we had been standing vacantly in front of the mirror for about two minutes while thinking about letters. To be vain is an awful thing. We said 'I'm not looking at me,' but it was too late. Trish thinks we are self-obsessed and will probably tell everyone.

At 9.01am, we hear the invigilator say 'You may start now.'

But of course, we may not start.

We may not start until 9.41, which is how long it takes to sort everything. The official exam ends at 10.30, at which point the chairs squeal outward again as the majority of students in the room leave the hall. Outside the door we hear a swelling roar of postexam chat, unsuccessfully quashed by invigilators calling out 'SHHHHH, the exam isn't over for everyone!'

There is something calming about a room that is intended to hold a lot of people being empty, or in this case, relatively empty—nine of us are left. It's like a theatre after the performance when everyone has shuffled out, and all the adrenaline has evaporated because it no longer serves any purpose. The room is silent apart from the soft flicking of pages—the others are checking through their papers. The only constant sound is our own pen scribbling; we're writing so furiously we would not be surprised if when our exam paper gets taken away, the tracks of everything we wrote were inscribed on the desk. In this last half an hour, blissfully, we manage to finish the paper, adding the word <u>G</u>EEK to our list to account for anyone who noticed us scribbling away madly.

Afterwardss we leave the room with Alice, a fellow Extra Timer.

'How did it go?' we try.

'Shit,' she replies, swigging from her water bottle. 'Why do you even get Extra Time anyway? It's so unfair, because you're really clever.'

'I'm a slow processor.'

'What does that even mean? It sounds totally made up.'

This is hard to dispute.

Lying scummy cheat.
Lying scummy cheat.
Lying scummy cheat.

The rest of our GCSEs pass in a similarly uncomfortable fashion, but despite my moaning, I would be happy for them to drag on forever. The end of GCSEs will signal the end of this phase of school life. The junior-school days will be over, and we'll move out of Wimborne and into Austen, an ugly prefab bungalow on the outskirts of the school grounds, which looks like it replaced something that got bombed in the war, except that it didn't.

Girls going into sixth form are allowed to make a list of a few people they want to be in a house with. We and Scarlett held an emergency conference on the fire escape connecting Wimborne and Aylingforde and engineered our lists so that we'd be certain to end up together, along with Ellie. We and Alice won't be in the same house, because all our friends outside Wimborne are different. Georgia is leaving to go to a different school, where she can focus more on her running.

It's not a major deal who you end up with really, because everyone in sixth form gets their own room so they can revise for their A-levels. This means there will be no one to distract us from the monotony of the letters.

She will relish this opportunity to have long evenings and nights to ourselves, analysing our data. She will say that now we have our own room, it's better to avoid people altogether, because our bad behaviour only generates more words and creates more routines.

She is about to take hold, and there is nothing that I can do about it.

12

Coming Home

In Wimborne everyone tacked pictures round their beds, and my collection has grown steadily over three years. I cart them over to Austen and stick them up: a Technicolor wallpaper of photos, concert tickets, postcards, and pages ripped from magazines. Most importantly, an assortment of paper notes I've saved with cute messages on them from Georgia and Ellie— handwritten proof of a stellar performance that sold out every night these last three years, though no one ever knew it was happening.

LILY—Can we go for a run later? I loveeee you! Lilz you are the best and I'm so lucky to have you as my friend. Xxxx

I have my same crepe flower chains, same spotty duvet cover, same—

Oh, but it isn't the same. Lessons finished at 3.00pm today, and we came straight back here. We dumped our folders and patent pencil case on the desk, and then the door shut behind us with a soft click. The other voices in the corridor went out like lights, but that was when the bomb went off.

You took me straight to:

CBKCTHSTGMFLSPDLIAGCSHQO.
CBKCTHSTGMFLSPDLIAGCSHQO.
CBKCTHSTGMFLSPDLIAGCSHQO.

You took me there, sat rigid on the end of the bed for hours and hours, and might have kept me there forever were it not that it's 7.00pm now, which means it's time for roll call.

We resurface from our room and paste a neutral expression over our face. Girls upon girls are cramming into the common room in small groups; the noise of their conversations all at once is a jungle sound track with no way in. A group of sofas face our new housemaster, Mr Elingham, who stands at the front of the room, waiting to tick names off a sheet.

There's nowhere left to sit! But then, thank god, we see Ellie and Scarlett, scooting apart from each other on the sofa and patting an opening between them. We walk over and perch there, panic brewing because our knees are touching theirs.

Whoooosh! A girl called Stephanie zooms in. 'Make way!' she calls, throwing herself upon us and lying sprawled there with her bum on our lap and her shoulders and head in Scarlett's arms. The feeling of her on top of us is overwhelming; she's a giant burbling baby in our arms. Our faces are too close. We are certain she smells something on our breath, our body; here comes another girl, pauses to look down at us, arms akimbo in faux outrage at the lack of space, before laughing. 'Budge up!'—

(Girls upon
girls upon
girls upon
girls)

We stink! There are too many of us on this sofa, and they all know—

Scarlett nudges us, turning a dial and twizzling us back in from between stations. Mr Elingham is looking at us expectantly.

Argh! She revs. *Tsk tsk, what a little freak you are! Don't you know your own name when it's called?*

'Yes?' we answer. He gives us a warm smile, ticks the paper, and continues down the list before starting to read out notices. I sit through it, trying not to do anything that will make her even angrier. It finally ends, Stephanie pushes off, and She marches me back to my room before Ellie and Scarlett can get in the way.

The mirror nailed to the wall is confronting.

A face stares back, but I can't call it my own. I place my hands on either side of it and open my mouth to scream. I am not brave enough to make noise, but I open my mouth wider and watch my nose scrunch itself into a dragon snout, my eyes squeezing into slits. I didn't know it was possible to shout on mute, but it is.

I open and close my mouth:

Arrrrrrrrghhh!

Then I pull the skin on my cheeks down hard, so the fleshy salmon rims of my lower eyelids flip outward. There's me, finally seen as I should be, twisted into something as monstrous as I feel.

Whhhhhhhhy, I mouth. *Whhhhhhhhy?*

WHAT ARE YOU DOING? She yells. *This behaviour is the height of vanity.*

I drop to the floor. It suddenly seems essential that I make myself as small as possible.

I don't care, I say. *I don't care what happens anymore as long as it doesn't involve letters and lists.*
I want to die. There. Are you happy?
I just want it to end.

It's my idea, I said it first. But She seizes it and moulds it into her own shape. I feel her seep into my arms, her grip supplanting mine.

So we're in agreement. We can't go on like this. We need to be somewhere that doesn't involve interactions with people day in, day out. It's making you so unhappy, poor thing. We'll fix it. But we need to work together on this. Because we're on the same team.
Aren't we?

If you want to come home from boarding school, you have to be sick. Crying doesn't do it. Neither does lying in bed.

We can do sickness.

We make our throat raspy and throw up a few times. We do star jumps and put a hot water bottle to our head until we are over 38°C.

'Gosh, you are hot,' says Matron, clicking her tongue, and then, a little later: 'Your mother's just called.' She rearranges the wet flannel on our head and smooths down the covers.

'She's on her way now to get you.'

Mum makes it in under two hours. She picks us up and chucks our bag in the trunk, and we whir down country lanes in silence.

Then she breaks it—smash—100,000,000 shards—exploding nebulas of words and words and words—

'What the hell is the matter with you anyway?'

We hit a pothole, and the car stalls. The radio we hadn't realised was on shuts up momentarily and rebounds like one of those annoying dolls with the weight in their bottom so they can't topple over.

'I don't know. Can we get something to eat?'

'Yes.'

We pull over at the next petrol station.

'Do you want to get out?'

We shake our head.

'Well, what do you want then?'

While she's inside, some men in a white van pull up. They are ogling us like there is no one inside our head to notice. We worry that we might get pregnant with their child as a punishment for letting them look when we should be charging out of the car and screaming in defence of feminism, so we give them the finger. They honk.

We sit shivering in our parka. Mum appears, running across the tarmac through sheets of rain made neon against the dark by car headlamps, shielding her hair with her arm and darting between the pumps. She passes us a plastic bag containing Jammie Dodgers biscuits and raspberries.

'Thanks.'

We eat in silence and listen to the rustle of packaging on our lap and the chomping of jaws and temples.

It isn't much of a homecoming. Mum runs us a bath and watches us sit in it until the water goes cold. We hunch over our stubbly legs and offend her with our modesty. Then she brings us a scabby towel and looks away while we stand up, dripping suds, waiting to get wrapped up like a newborn.

In the morning we seek advice from the herbal therapist who lives in our town. His name is Monty, and we are told that he is well respected by the homeopathic community. Mum loves his shop and treats him with a level of respect befitting a brain surgeon.

She explains that we are feeling blue. We are embarrassed, but Mum says, 'It's okay, we can trust this man, he knows lots about medicine and how to make people like you feel better. He just wants to ask you a few questions.'

'Do you study biology, Lily? Do you understand about the importance of maintaining healthy mineral levels in the blood, Lily?' He has a thick South African accent. We wish he would stop saying our name like he knows us.

'I used to study it, but I dropped it for A-level.'

'When exactly did you become sick?'

'I don't know that I—'

'Fever?'

'Sorry?'

'Shaky? Clammy? Wake up in the night in a hot sweat—take off all your clothes, only to find yourself shivering 15 minutes later and reaching for a pair of thick socks?'

'Doesn't everyone?'

'How do you feel right now?'

'Tired.'

'How often do you stool?'

Pause.

'I have a chair in my room. I'm not sure?'

Apparently this is not the right answer. People laugh. He gives us hippie pills that come in old-fashioned-looking glass brown bottles with gold lids. They will rebalance our energy levels and make us feel better.

Thanking him, Mum ushers us back into the car. Glancing back, we see him doing some sort of farewell Buddha bow from the window.

On Tuesday Mum takes us to the GP, who measures our blood pressure and sends us off for iron and thyroid gland hormone testing. We go to the local walk-in centre with a long doctor's scrawl of things lab technicians need to search for in our body.

A spiky-haired Hungarian nurse jabs at our arm a few times, struggling to find a vein. A doddery old man with slack lips and a drooly chin leers in at us through a crack in the curtain. The nurse slaps a shiny bravery sticker we are too old for on our shirt. The truth is, we are 16 now. If she knew, would she have taken the sticker back? She says to call back in a few days' time if we haven't heard.

After that we spend the next few days in bed, lying as still as possible because it's easier not to do things wrong this way. The GP calls on Friday to say the levels of everything in our body are fine.

'A bit low on iron. You could take supplements if you like. It probably wouldn't make much difference. It's a personal choice. Talk to your mother about it.'

School phones too. 'Is Lily coming back soon?' Something about Sunday night and everyone needing a bit of a rest sometimes. Mum hangs up. She comes to tell us, but we pad away from where our ear has been against the door and rush back into bed. We pretend to be asleep. Our heart beats fast, racing with deceit.

FAKED SLEEP: We lied in that we faked sleep, but it was acceptable. We needed to avoid speaking to Mum until composure had been resumed.

Sunday comes around too fast. All too soon we are back in the car headed for school, leaving London behind, fleeing lampposts, surrendering light and traffic for hedgerows and the moon.

'You'll have to see the school doctor,' says our housemaster, a few hours after Mum has gone.

Mr Elingham has only been our housemaster for a few weeks, but we can tell he has already mentally picked us out as being a potentially problematic pupil. This is probably partly because in the first week we were in Austen, he caught us going through the bin in the middle of the night like a deranged posh girl playing a hobo.

We were doing this because we had become worried that we might have thrown away a piece of paper with highly incriminating information on it, without actually remembering the act of throwing it away. We were gripped by the urge to root around in the bin and make sure we hadn't, so that no one was able to use the information to destroy our life.

Only Mr Elingham didn't know that. He just stood there wide-eyed and startled, as if his teacher training hadn't prepared him properly. We were startled too. We dropped the banana skin between our thumb and forefinger and whizzed our hands behind our back in the hope that he wouldn't notice our latex gloves. We stuttered an excuse about having lost something, but we could tell he didn't buy it.

'I'm not ill,' we reply.

'You missed a week of school. In my book that counts as unwell—'

'I was tired—'

'I've booked you in for four o'clock on Tuesday.'

'I don't want to go.'

'No one's writing you a prescription, no one's saying anything serious. You missed a week of school, and now you have to go to one 30-minute appointment. In my book that's a small price to pay. Don't you think?'

Mr Elingham has a lot of stupid ideas in his book.

It's Tuesday, 4.37pm. Two younger students have gone in already: one with a sprained ankle and the other with a tummy ache.

She says:

Whatever you do, do not mention me.

'I hope you don't mind,' Tess the school nurse whisper-shouts across the waiting room, 'we just have to make sure the sick folks get seen first.'

We're waiting for an hour.

Who cares? says my friend.

I care, I say.

We backward-flip through July's *Teen Vogue* and *Glamour*. Across from us, pamphlets in a rack advertise the best treatment for various common ailments, like in a real doctor's office instead of this private-school attempt at one.

'Lol. I have neither of those, innit,' says a spotty girl with big boobs in the year above, pointing at leaflets about safe sex and skin cancer. 'Should that make me happy or sad man?' She turns to her friend in search of the recognition her joke deserves.

'Both,' the friend assents. 'It means you're cray, and you got your whole life ahead of you. Ya know what I'm saying bruv?'

Why do the children of the rich insist on talking like this? It makes us mad.

We look out the window and carry on with our lists.

'The doctor will see you now,' calls Tess. Dr Ford has a lazy eye and frumpy jeans, but something about her is liberating.

So I tell her, tell her the secret. Not all of it.

She is screaming:

Leave me out.
Leave me out.
Leave me OUT!

So I don't tell Dr Ford about us. I simply say that I make lists about things, day and night, and that I can't stop it.

I don't talk for long, maybe 45 seconds, just long enough to get the basics out. Dr Ford listens quietly and nods encouragingly. When I'm finished, she looks at me expectantly for a few seconds, as if she's waiting for something else. What is she waiting for? She pushes a box of tissues towards me.

Oh, that.

'I'm not much of a crier,' I say.

Dr Ford tells me I may have a mental health problem ('Because I didn't cry?' 'No, because of what you said before you didn't cry'), and then she mentions a different patient who had to stay up all night knitting, or she thought bad things would happen. This doesn't really sound like what I have, but I nod because I don't want to be rude. She says I have to see a specialist.

Dr Ford refers us to Dr Finch, who we are about to see for the first time.

My friend does not like the idea of Dr Finch.

Dr Finch practices in a hospital half an hour from school, and Mum drives from London to Kent to take us.

We plummet down topsy-turvy roads with the sunlight flash-flashing through the hedgerows.

She is restless. She thrashes about like a small child in uncomfortable lace clothing.

We turn left and enter the—

PSYCHIATRIC HOSPITAL

13

Doctor, Doctor

A woman swings round the doorway to the waiting room. She wears a long skirt and has puffy strawberry-blonde hair. 'Lily?' she says, like our name is a question in itself. 'Lily?'

I want to resent her for it, but I don't. Perhaps she is so intelligent, she doesn't have to use full sentences when she meets someone. She is a doctor, after all. And a woman. It's hard to be both. They say it isn't anymore, but the truth is, it is. We still haven't looked up. We probably should. 'Lily?'

Mum sighs, exasperated. 'Lily is over here,' she says, poking us.

Standing up is hard—She has flown down into our legs and oscillates with vengeance, knotting threads only I can see round the chair legs. Mum stays where she is, magazine on lap, reading but not reading, and we finally get up and follow Dr Finch. Her office is tucked away at the top of the building, along a reassuringly out-of-the-way corridor. She says to sit down, so we do, and we watch her shut the door and arrange herself on the chair opposite us with a file on her lap.

'Tell me about you,' she says.

I squeeze my eyes shut and try to hold on to this moment. These short few seconds are the bridge between when then becomes now. Then: you and me, together and on a mission to make me perfect, wedded together by our shared purpose. Now:

a secret told that can't be unspoken, a bond broken beyond repair thanks to my weakness. Everything I know about my world so far, changed by what I say next.

The promise of a full confession was made when I told Dr Ford the first part, even if I didn't know it at the time. The facts are hard but irrefutable: I don't want to live like this anymore. And any second now, I am going to tell the truth:

'There are two of me in my head.'

Something strange has happened.

My head feels clear and fresh, like being dunked in an ice bucket and pulled out by the scruff of your neck—or slapped across the face by someone you respect.

These thoughts that have plagued me don't define me.

These rules that must be obeyed to make sure nothing goes wrong might just be the things messing everything up.

'Was she helpful?' Mum asks tentatively, cutting through steak and kidney pie in the pub where we've gone for a debrief.

'Yes—in a way. I have obsessive-compulsive disorder, but it's treatable.'

'Why didn't you tell me?'

'I didn't know. I'd heard of OCD, but I thought it was all about lining up your books and checking the door's locked. I mean, I do have that door thing a bit, but it's so far from the main problem. . . . I didn't make the link.'

She squeezes my hand and bites her lip.

'I feel so terrible.'

'Why?'

'For not noticing.'

'You couldn't have. I live my life trying to come across as normal. All my energy seems to go into making sure no one *does* notice anything at all. If you knew, that would have meant I'd failed.'

'I don't get it, though. How is that OCD? I'm not saying I don't believe you fully—I do. But why don't I see you doing things over and over?'

'I do it all in my head.' I stop. I don't want to talk to her about it properly; it was bad enough with a stranger. The whole thing is so shameful and exposing; it's the naked-in-public nightmare, apart from the good bit where you wake up. And yet, of everyone who I could possibly tell, I think she probably deserves to know the most.

'Darling?'

'I make lists in my head of everything I've done that might be wrong. Then I repeat them over and over again and analyse them. I have to be perfect. I feel like if I do this enough, then one day I will be.'

'Why?'

'Why what?'

'Why do you have to be perfect?'

'You know what?' I smile properly for the first time in days. 'I've never really thought about it.'

My head is my own for two hours: no lists, no nothing. It is eerily quiet. I imagine myself bobbing about in a nighttime sea, alone on a small boat with no destination or guiding stars.

My friend doesn't like this.

Don't think She won't put up a fight.

She will.

She will tell me that I can't cope without her; that I will do crazy things; that I will be irresponsible. And She will say that—

people will watch you, but you won't remember how to smile. When you open your mouth to say 'I agree, we should go to lessons, I'll just get my pencil case,' what you'll actually snarl is 'Fuck you, little bitch.'

No conversations will ever be the same, because without me to regulate things, you'll become a bully. A mean, selfish waste of a soul. A manipulator.

You'll be the girl who makes other girls cry in the toilet. The girl who destroys the weakest one in the room—a cat swinging a mouse in its teeth, not for survival, just for fun—

I hate Dr Finch for taking something away, even temporarily.

It is 7.35pm. We are sitting cross-legged on our bed, staring hard at the wall. Anger is coming. At first it's just a rumbling on the horizon, like distant horses coming over the hill, but it draws closer, becoming bigger and bigger . . . the swords are in view, glinting in the low evening sun, and the horses don't look like toys anymore. They are almost life-size, getting more real and . . .

She and I have a conversation:

Have I ever let you down?

In what way?

You have friends. You are liked. Okay, you're not the most popular girl in the school, but you're above average. You have a personality. You have a character. You are not a blank space of nothingness like you always feared. When you do things wrong, we put them right. So, tell me: Why did you tell? Have I ever let you down?

No, yes. No. Well, not really. It's just . . . sometimes I wonder, does it have to be this hard? Maybe if we didn't try to remember everything and make it right, things would still be okay? I know you look after me. But for the last few years I've been in so much pain. I've been wondering if there's an easier way.

You only think that because you've seen some snotty psychiatrist who claims she can make you better. Well, she can't. She doesn't know you. Not like me. And she never will. Think how many patients she sees a day. You're just one of many fucked-up people she gets paid to pretend to like. What does she know about anything? You're safer with me. And you better not tell her about me. If you do, she'll think you're nuts, kaput, crazy—it's a one-way ticket to the madhouse. Do you understand? Keep your mouth shut.

From now on, Mum drives up from London every week, to take us to see Dr Finch at Fieldness Hospital. The sessions are arranged to be during free periods, and that way we don't miss any classes. The whole thing is kept hush-hush. Mr Elingham knows where we go, but he is very discreet, and says it's fine for Mum to take me out of school once a week for as long as is needed. I was wrong to think he was interfering. He really does just want the best for me. He checks in—asks me how I am.

On Thursdays, we wait in my room for Mum to call and let us know she's arrived. When she does, we check the coast is clear before legging it out to her car in the Austen forecourt. She'll be sitting in her silver Beetle, slunk low in her seat, wearing giant paparazzi-proof sunglasses. We have given her clear instructions. 'Be totally inconspicuous. Under no circumstances talk to anyone.'

We dive into the passenger seat. 'Drive!' we shout. 'Drive!'

She accelerates, and away we go. The drive out runs past the main building, and we really could see anyone. Teachers going between lessons, other girls walking back to their houses . . . We are desperate not to.

Mum gets it, and she assumes the role of the getaway driver. A shiny battalion of girls from our year rise up on the right, canvas book bags swinging, legs in sync as they march across the green. We duck. 'TAKE COVER!' yells Mum. 'Get down!' Our head is in our lap. We feel the rumble of tarmac beneath me hum through our body.

'As you were!' She laughs, impersonating an officer. 'They're gone.'

It takes up half her day, coming here and back. But she never complains.

Dr Finch's first job is to convince us that we do actually have OCD. We are not sold. In particular, my friend has grievances. She says:

OCD is a mental disorder. Mental disorder implies bad. What we do is good. It's helpful, constructive, and without it you wouldn't know who you were or how to be consistent. Okay, so it got a little out of hand.

Perhaps we were sometimes recording some stuff that didn't need to be recorded.

We can go easier in the future.

We can let some things slide.

I am quite certain this is not OCD.

'Okay,' says Dr Finch. 'I am sure you have OCD. In fact, it's been a very long time since I saw someone so young with OCD as progressed as yours. But as most people think it always relates to cleaning or straightening things or being meticulously organised, it's not surprising that you don't think you have OCD. So let's take a step back and look at what OCD is.

'Obsessions are recurring thoughts and images that cause you distress. You don't want to have them, but you can't stop them coming, and it's hard to make them go away. In your case, you obsess over things you think you've done wrong.

'Compulsions are the things you repeatedly do in response to the obsessions. In your case, you make lists in your head of things you've done wrong and go through each word, trying to make it better.

'Doing compulsions is called neutralising. You can think of it as an attempt to 'cancel out' the obsession.'

I am beginning to feel a little more convinced.

She is sulking in a corner of my brain.

Remembering and analysing what we have done wrong improves our mood for a while, Dr Finch says. 'But the problem is that in the long term, going along with your compulsions just increases the frequency of the obsessions. So you get this vicious circle going on, where the more you try to avoid anxiety, the more anxious you become.

'I'm going to draw it for you.'

She draws a line that wiggles up and down like a snake.

'This is what happens when you do a compulsion. Your anxiety initially goes down, but very soon after, it rockets back up again. So then you do another compulsion to get it back down, but then bam, more obsessions, and it goes back up. You get the idea.'

She draws another line. At first, this one goes higher than the first line, but then it gradually starts going down again, until it's lower than the lowest point on the first line.

'And this is what happens when you resist a compulsion.

Initially, your anxiety soars higher than it would if you just did the compulsion. But then over time it comes back down to base level and eventually goes lower than it would by doing a compulsion. And because you're resisting the compulsions, it doesn't go back up.'

'So what you're saying is that if I don't want to feel so bad, I shouldn't record the words and analyse them? I shouldn't react to them when they pop into my head?'

'Yes. That is exactly what I'm saying.'

This thought is as startling as a bullet hitting me from behind.

'How would you feel about taking medication?'

We are prescribed fluoxetine: Prozac. We had no idea Prozac was used to treat anything apart from depression, but it turns out it is also used for people with OCD. Our dose will go up every few weeks, and eventually we will be taking about three times as much as someone with depression.

Fluoxetine is dispensed to the school, and we pick it up from the med centre. In the nurses' office, Tess squints over her glasses and hands us the pills, pinching her lips into a prune. We can tell she is itching to ask 'What fucked you up, then? Look at this lovely school you go to. What gives you the right to be unhappy?'

At first, we don't notice much. But after a few weeks, the pills make us tired and groggy. I start to care less about everything. Friends, family, and, crucially, routines.

She is calling for me to engage with her, but She feels distant, like a voice echoing from the top of a wooded hill. I try to keep up with the routines but cannot muster the mental energy to do as much in-depth analysis with her.

Our memory also seems to be worsening. Occasionally letters slip away, or the letter is remembered but not the accompanying word. We've started writing the letters on our skin so they are not forgotten. They wind their way around our left hand and down our fingers, before crawling up our arm like spiders.

She stomps around. She is cranky and bitchy.

She moans:

You're killing me. After all I've done for you. You're poisoning me with those orange and green pills. You could hang me, but you don't have the guts. So instead you've opted for a long and drawn-out death.

Well, fine. Have it your way.

But I won't go quietly.

14

Pills, Pills, Pills

It turns out that having a friend is uncommon.

'But then,' says Dr Finch, 'some people do say they hear their OCD as a voice. . . . It's difficult to know exactly how someone's OCD feels unless you're actually in their head. It could be because you had OCD from when you were so young that it was just easier for you to see it that way.'

She wants to discuss the obsession about being a bad person.

'We're going to look at something called Theory A and Theory B. I'll draw it for you.'

She writes Theory A in the first of two columns and Theory B in the second. She writes a message under each heading and hands us the paper. Her writing is thin and messy.

'Which do you think you are?' asks Dr Finch.

'Theory A.'

Theory A is:

I am a bad person, and I must do everything possible to record everything bad that I do.

Theory B is:

The problem is not that I am a bad person, but that I am excessively worried about being a bad person.

'Okay. Well, in order to get you better, we need to do CBT,

cognitive behavioural therapy. In OCD, a key element of CBT is exposure and response prevention, known as exposure therapy.

'You're going to have to repeatedly sit with your obsessions without doing a compulsion—putting them on your list and analysing them to make them go away.

'Over time, practicing this healthy behaviour is going to make it automatic. Because your compulsions take up so much of your day, you're going to be doing constant exposure therapy.'

So I try acting like Theory B is right. When I accidentally glance at the body of a girl in a lower grade, I attempt to act as though the problem is not that someone will think I am a pervert, the problem is that I *worry* too much that someone will think I am a pervert.

When our tummy rumbles or I end up scratching our nose without thinking about it, I try to believe that I am not disgusting and everyone knows it, I am just worrying too much about ordinary things.

I try to let letters come—and not respond to them.

TOILET: We came out the toilet, and Ellie was waiting outside the door to use it. We'd only done a pee, but suddenly we felt like we had done a huge shit and it was all over the whole toilet, the walls and the floor. We needed to go back and check. We couldn't do that because that would look weird. We froze. Ellie raised an eyebrow. Did this whole interaction look odd? Was there actually shit everywhere?

Don't respond to it. Don't engage with it. Ignore the letter— And guess what? I can't. None of it.

Can't do it. Won't do it.

Dr Finch is not disappointed. I tell her there has probably been about a five percent improvement, but that I think it is mostly down to the medication, because I haven't been very successful at resisting doing the compulsions.

'That's okay,' she says. 'It's not going to happen overnight. And five percent is a great start, since you've only been coming to see me for a few weeks. I feel quite positive about five percent.'

She parrots in a baby voice:

'A great start! I feel quite positive! Go get 'em! Everyone's a winner! Psychiatry rocks!'

I stifle a laugh.

'Sometimes I feel like there's two people in the room sitting opposite me,' Dr Finch says, 'having a conversation about me, and I have absolutely no idea what they are saying.'

Dr Finch gives me homework, and I have to report back to her when I next see her. This week I am supposed to interrupt our routines, and keep doing it until I can't remember them anymore. This means every time we find a Pause and start doing a routine, I should snap out of it and do something else instead.

'Your routines feed off isolation,' says Dr Finch. 'During breaks, when you would usually go back to your dorm and lie on your bed to do routines, have a break. Go to the canteen, get a cup of tea, sit with your friends.

'Even if you're not actively chatting, just being there takes you away from all that time in your room on your own. If it's the evening and you're sitting in your room by yourself doing routines, go and knock on Scarlett's door. You've told me before how close you are. I'm sure she would want to help.' So far, Dr Finch has only given me one task per week, but this week she sets two. For the second, we talk about the way everything is done in threes. Hand washing, light switches, and locking doors are the visible tip of an otherwise fully submerged iceberg. *Tap, invert, sleeves,* and *hair* are noticeable, but only to an attuned eye. The rest, the rhythmic repetition of letters, thoughts, and actions . . . how could anyone guess?

Dr Finch asks which of these things would be hardest to give up. I tell her: thoughts. Not that the others will be easy.

'Okay,' she starts. 'We're going to do graded exposure. We'll start with whatever you find least intimidating and work our way up to the hardest. So the physical things. Because we need to do something about those hands.'

I look at my lap.

My sleeves are pulled down as far as possible to cover my hands, but the knuckles are visible. Red and scaly, rippling like the back of a Chinese dragon. Peeling, scabby.

Raw to the bone.

I don't think about them too much. In the back of my mind, I am aware that they are very painful when they are moved or brushed against, like they have been held forcibly over a fire, but She turns the discomfort down like a dimmer switch.

Dr Finch wonders how many times a day I'm washing them. 'About 50.'

'And every time you wash them, you do it three times? With three lots of soap?'

'Yes.'

At what point did all this start?

We think it was the advert on TV for antibacterial sprays and soaps where dirt is seen in ultraviolet light, infecting everywhere.

I kill 99.9 percent of dirt! Buy me!

But what about the 0.01 percent? we are screaming. *What about the 0.01 percent?*

Or the things Mum and Dad told us—germs are bad, sometimes you can't see them, bacteria spreads disease; remember cleanliness. The things all parents say.

'Okay. So if we could get you only washing them once each time, that's already a lot less. Let's do an exposure.'

Dr Finch leads us to the bathroom down the hall. Under her instruction, we turn on the tap and wash our hands once. Knowing we are not going to do it twice more makes our heart catch and beat faster; we feel like we are burning from the inside out.

My friend reasons that this is just a stupid experiment, and it doesn't have to count if we don't want it to. We take three paper towels from the dispenser, using one to turn the tap off (so we don't have to touch it with our 33.33 percent recurring clean hands) and the other two to dry our hands. Dr Finch notices and says

'Mess it up. Take another one.'

'What?'

'Feel uncomfortable with the number. Take four paper towels.'

'But that's even more?'

'When we're doing exposure about numbers, it's so ingrained that sometimes you're going to do stuff in threes without even thinking. When that happens, it's easy to say 'Oh, I've failed, never mind,' but actually there's still the opportunity to do an exposure by just going a number higher: it's still the 'wrong' number of times, right? I'm using this opportunity to show you how to do it.'

We're not paying attention. We are busy thinking.

One soap squirt + four paper towels = five.

Five is a bad number, and we don't like it one bit.

I write notes in a little blue book with spirals on the front.
SUCCESSES:

1. I went to first break four out of five times this week. People were talking, so I couldn't review routines, and full review was put off until lunchtime, when I went back to my dorm. Along the way, so much piled up that I forgot what some letters stood for. I haven't managed to retrieve them.

2. On Friday, Ellie came into my dorm at lunch and started an in-depth dissection of the character flaws of her boyfriend Ben. She stayed for 45 minutes, until it was time for class. We walked to the main building together. About 20 percent of the letters slipped away.

3. I have switched off lights and plugs only once, but I am so used to doing everything in threes that I usually forget at first and have to go up to a higher number like four or five.
The same goes for passing my hand under taps in multiples of three to check that I can't feel water coming out and that my eyes aren't deceiving me.

4. When I wash my hands only once, She tells me that I will have dirty smears left on my fingers, which I will spread to everything I touch; that I will get hepatitis or AIDS and give it to others; that

not doing things three times will cause Mum to be in an accident or Ella to be unhappy at school or Tuffy to get hit by a car. Her threats change so fast, it's difficult to keep up.

According to Dr Finch, linking how many times you do something to bad things happening is an unhealthy behaviour done by lots of people with OCD. It's called magical thinking: where you believe you can control outcomes through your actions, even though you can't. So I keep reminding myself that magical thinking is a waste of time.

Mum can't take us to Fieldness today, so we get a taxi from school. Knowing Mum's not in the waiting room downstairs emboldens me to confess something.

I tell Dr Finch: 'There's something I haven't told you.'

'Go on.'

'I think I'm a psychopath.'

'Why?'

'I have this thought.'

'What's the thought?'

'I . . .' I try to tell her, but She won't let the words go.

She'll section you. She'll report you to the police. Don't say anything. This is not a thought to be shared with others.

'I can't do it.'

If you tell her, I'll leave.

'Try me.'

I mean it.

'No, honestly. This won't be something you've dealt with. I've heard that people with OCD tend to be caring. You'll be disgusted.'

'Try me.'

'I worry . . . I . . . My mum's best friend has cancer. And I can't stop thinking that I want her to die.'

The words come out in a rush. I expect her to push a panic button under her chair and for security guards to storm the room. I haven't even told her about the other thoughts:

I'm going to stab people in the dorms next to me while they are asleep.
I'm going to push Ella into the road.
I want my family to be in a car crash.

'Do you really want her to die?'

'No! That's the last thing I want. That's why I'm so upset that I can't stop thinking I want her to die.'

'So then that's it. It's a random horrible thought that pops into your head, an intrusive thought. Everyone in the population sometimes has intrusive thoughts. Someone who has OCD is more likely to think they are hugely significant and ruminate about them.'

She gets up and rummages through some papers on her desk, before finding a printout of a list headed 'Common Intrusive Thoughts.' It's quite a list:

Thought that you might jump off a bridge or into the road
Thought that you may 'lose control' and start attacking someone
Thought of a sexual nature about someone inappropriate such as a family member or a child

Thought that goes against your sexual preference

Thought of doing something inappropriate in a religious place

Thought that you may have committed a crime you have read about

Thought of an authority figure naked

Thought that you are going to start swearing in public

Thought that you want someone, particularly a loved one, to die

'Healthy people get these thoughts. Most people have thought at a train station: 'What if I pushed the person next to me on the track?' But when someone without OCD gets that thought, they just think 'Oh, that was weird, that's not me at all,' and get on with their life. A lot of the time they probably don't even remember it. It's a total non-event. Someone like you has a different reaction.'

How can it be that the dark thoughts She said made me uniquely evil are just a characteristic of an illness?

I am torn between feeling frustrated that I didn't know this before, and utterly relieved that I am not a dangerous person.

I need clarification. Not being able to stop these thoughts doesn't make people with OCD evil and dangerous?

'On the contrary,' says Dr Finch. 'The reason people with OCD find these thoughts so upsetting is because they are so completely at odds with their values. The problem with people who have OCD is that they care too much. They are some of the safest people in the world. No one with OCD has ever acted on an intrusive thought, nor will they.'

'But what if someone with intrusive thoughts goes to a doctor who doesn't know much about OCD and thinks they are a psychopath?'

'That can and does happen if the professional doesn't have any experience of OCD. But most can usually tell it's obviously not that, just from the amount of anxiety the person in front of them is attaching to the thoughts. Some psychopaths have these thoughts too, but they mean them and are not made anxious by them. For them it's not a fearful thought. It's something they actually want to do. The difference is paramount.'

'How can I stop it?'

'When the thought comes,' says Dr Finch, 'don't push it away. That will make it worse. Just think 'Oh, look. It's that thought again. It doesn't mean anything. It's not me.' Don't attach significance to it. If it loses its power to be scary, it won't hurt you anymore.'

We run overtime. We are late for the taxi, and the driver in the courtyard is cross.

Our breath sticks in our throat like we have swallowed a fly. We hate it when people get angry. Dr Finch has come out too, which she doesn't usually do. She puts her hand on my back.

'I'm sorry,' she tells the driver, 'it's my fault. I kept her longer than I should have.' Then she turns to us. 'See you next week.'

I should say something, anything. Stutter good-bye or something. A thank-you. But I don't know how. She put her hand on my back!

She has turned already.

She's walking back, typing in the code, going through the door, oh god please turn around, please turn around, PLEASE TURN AROUND, even though she won't, she'll keep on walking, it meant nothing, she'll see you next week, between now and then she won't know who you are and—

'Are you coming or not? I have another job to get to.'

'Sorry. Fenhurst station.'

15

Driving

The noise wakes me. I find myself by the window, staring out, fat-eyed, into the night. There are no stars.

She has left me, I know, and is outside. I expect to see her crouched low in the bush beneath the windowsill, but She is not there.

So I wait, and begin to think maybe the knocking was only rain, and her whispering was just the rustling of trees outside. I decide She must be somewhere inside the house, and that I will go and look for her.

But just then, I see a wispy figure running into the distance. I know it's her, although it's strange, seeing her out of my head for the first time—I am so used to her sitting behind my eyes. Her feathery outline streaks in and out of the trees, and I jump out the window after her. For someone who's never used legs before, She is surprisingly good at it.

Eventually, there She is, sprawled under a big tree. I crawl in next to her, and ask her where She has been today. She doesn't talk to me anymore. She just looks at me, and shakes her head like it's time.

Oh, say it isn't time. I know that I betrayed you, that I told Dr Finch about the thoughts when you told me never to say, but worse, the final insult—I've started to really like her.

I can't help myself. I want you both.

We lie, looking up to the moonless blue. It is raining, and we are drenched to our bones, our breath momentarily catching in our throats, feeling like sinking ships on a black ocean with no land in sight, and no stars because they all exploded and then died for good 100,000 years ago.

Why won't you hold my hand?
Come back.
Please.

I wake up without her. I go through the motions—breakfast, assembly, classes—but it's like tiptoeing through a city at dawn. I'm by myself on vast empty streets too quiet to seem real.

I don't do my lists all morning, but then I start to feel guilty and scared. If I don't do them just because She's not there to keep track, how will I know what kind of person I am?

I force myself to do my lists alone. It's harder than I thought.

She'll be back soon. She has to be. Doesn't she?

I once overheard someone on the train tell the girl she was sitting with that she went to a funeral and got the giggles. She got them badly. So badly she had to take a minute outside. She couldn't explain it—not then, not now.

Grief, she said. It does the weirdest things to you.

So maybe that's why, despite everything, I find myself in the Austen communal kitchen with Ella and Scarlett, dancing to 'Cotton Eye Joe' pumped up to full volume. We are spinning, twisting, and do-si-doing. We make manic clockwork figures of eight round the room.

> *If it hadn't been for Cotton Eye Joe*
> *I'd been married a long time ago*
> *Where did you come from, where did you go?*
> *Where did you come from, Cotton Eye Joe?*

The verse repeats again and again—are those the only words in the whole song? The three of us shriek with laughter. We hitch our school skirts up and tie our shirts in cowboy knots . . .

And I forget briefly how lonely I am, until later, when I'm lying in my bed after midnight trying to order mountains of letters by myself, and I can't.

> *Why don't you see?* I howl. *I didn't want you to really go.*
> *All you had to do was be nice.*

Dr Finch collects me from the waiting room. She tells me to come and have a seat, which annoys me. As if I'm going to stand up for the whole hour. Ridiculous woman.

'How are things?' she asks. Calm, regular.

'She's gone.'

'Who's gone?'

'My friend.'

'Are you angry with me?'

Silence.

'It would be perfectly natural if you were. You might feel like I've taken something away from you.'

Silence.

'Are you?'

'I thought you were going to make me better. She's gone, and I've never felt more alone. You told me there was only room for one of us in my head, and that it had to be me, because I am the real one, and She is OCD. But you were wrong. She was more real than me. I hate you for it.'

'That's understandable.'

I want to say *Oh, for god's sake, I've just told you I hate you. React, you overprofessional clinical monster.* But I stay silent.

'You've done it yourself. You got rid of 'her.' But you could bring her back if you wanted—she's your creation. She's your OCD. You can do whatever you want with her.'

'NO.'

Silence.

'I didn't create her, She created me. She told me what to do—how to react to things. I'm nothing without her. She's gone to punish me for telling you too much.'

Oh, oh, oh. I cradle my own head because now there is no one else to.

'I am a blank space. I am not accounting for my actions. I am becoming inconsistent in my behaviour. I don't know who I am.'

She is waiting outside Dr Finch's office, snickering.

Be careful what you wish for.

She throws her head back, roars with laughter, and skips off down the corridor.

'Did you have a good session, darling?' Mum asks as we're driving back.

'Yeah,' I say. 'It was okay.'

She sighs, fingers drumming the steering wheel.

'Are you okay?' I ask.

'I'm fine.'

She's not.

'I just wish I knew how to help you more. I'll be honest, I feel like I don't really know much about what you're going through. I know you're talking to Dr Finch about it, but you don't talk to me about it. Every time I ask you, you go all distant.'

This is true. It's also intentional. I don't want Mum or Dad to know what it's really like in my head—I am a soldier on the frontline somewhere awful, rightly or wrongly, deciding that my family should be spared the true horrors of what I see.

I hold my secrets close. It's not that hard, really. Being away at boarding school is conducive to deception.

'You've got that book though, the one about dealing with OCD that Dr Finch recommended.'

'But that doesn't tell me about *you*.'

'I don't like talking about *me*,' I say.

She turns the radio on.

We have two lungs. We have two kidneys. We have two sides of our brain. Two arms. Two legs. Two ears. Two nostrils. Two lips, eyes, boobs, segments of heart, hands, feet, labia. Everything in ourselves is geared towards there being two of us in our head. Now I have no one to share my spare parts with.

So I hate Dr Finch (almost). But in the midst of all this hate, I don't stop going to my appointments, because without my friend there is no one, and at least Dr Finch is someone.

Every week she arrives in the waiting room, wearing a different shade of ankle-skimming skirt. 'Hello,' I say.

I am angry because in the beginning she said that if I wasn't happy when She had gone, she would bring her back. Now I realise that was just something she said to make me take part in her strategies. I also understand that it's not that she wouldn't bring her back—perhaps if she knew how unhappy I am, she would try. It's that she can't. My friend has departed of her own accord. What remains is a strange hollow; I am a twin left behind in a womb too big for only me. I try to talk to her; try to get her to help me with my lists, but there's no reply. My calls for her ring out into the void, where they stay, unanswered. So I carry out the routines by myself (*See, friend, I am your student, your diligent protégé, and I will continue your life's work*), but without her to supervise, it all feels wrong.

Today I tell Dr Finch my theory of twos.

'Yes'—she, usually so professional, wrings her hands in exasperation—'but we have ONE BODY.'

I am stunned.

She is in full flow.

'You know who your 'friend' reminds me of? A wife beater. She beats you up in your head and calls you names when you don't do what she says, and you follow her instructions because you're scared of all the supposed things she could make happen if you don't. And then, just when you're at your lowest point, she comes and wraps her arms round you and whispers reassuring things in your ear and you're persuaded into thinking she loved you all along. Her occasional niceness wins you over every time. You think none of the bad things will ever happen again, but they always do. I'm right, aren't I?'

I mope: 'But when I had her in my head, I didn't feel so lonely.'

Dr Finch has a suggestion. She blushes as she says it.

'Couldn't you put me in your head instead?'

'What?'

She seems genuinely embarrassed; her face goes a deep cherry red. 'Well, couldn't . . . When you have urges to give in to your rituals, or are feeling sad that your friend isn't there anymore, couldn't I be there instead?'

'I could never put you in my head. It's a terrible place for anyone to be—and I don't want you to be there.'

'But I wouldn't really be there. It would just be a model of me, so I wouldn't be feeling any pain.'

'But that's the other problem: if I can't have you for real, I don't want you at all.'

I am sitting in the back row in philosophy. At the front of the classroom, Mr Alan is presenting an introductory slideshow on Sigmund Freud.

I haven't been paying much attention. I am coming to the end of a series of words I've been focusing on for about 40 minutes, while staring at the tarmac path outside the window. It is so hot, it is turning into sticky black licorice. A fan whirs in the room. Suddenly Mr Alan says something that demands my full attention:

'Freud was the father of psychoanalysis. He believed that the origin of neuroses was sexual trauma.'

I cry out 'What?' as though I am personally outraged by what he has just said. I didn't mean to, it just came out. Ten ponytails swivel and replace themselves with pouty faces. Mr Alan raises his eyebrows at me. I don't usually ask questions. On the slide show, the words *repression*, *sexual abuse*, and *obsessional neurosis* are swelling. I worry they might escape the screen. My ears are buzzing.

'I'm just getting on to explaining it properly, Lily,' says Mr

Alan, 'if you'll let me continue. Freud's seduction theory was a hypothesis he formed in the 1890s. After studying a group of patients suffering from a range of nervous disorders, he realised the one thing they all had in common was that they had been sexually abused as children. He came to believe that a repressed memory of molestation or sexual abuse in childhood caused hysterical or obsessional symptoms.'

I cannot listen anymore. I ask to be excused and return to house. I sit at the end of my bed in my dorm with my head in my hands and my phone next to me. I wait for it to buzz to let me know Mum is here. It's Therapy Thursday, so she should be here soon.

Her car pulls up in the forecourt. I push the door buzzer to let myself out and hop into the front seat. 'Are you okay?' she says gently. 'You look like you've seen a ghost.'

'I don't wanna talk right now,' I say, knowing I am being unfair. She has driven all the way from London.

'Okay, darling,' she says, handing me a hummus sandwich and some Jammie Dodgers. 'Whatever you want.'

By the time I reach Dr Finch, I have worked myself into a state. It feels like I will never be calm again. As soon as I'm in her office, I tell her about Freud in a huge rush. I explain that when I was younger, I played a strange game—

No! Of course it wasn't with my mum or dad, or even anyone in my family. It was with a child, a little boy who I was close too. I used to play at his house, our parents were friends—

I ask if it was my fault and if I am bad. I ask her if this is why I am ill; is it true that this sort of thing causes obsessional symptoms?

Dr Finch says not to take much notice of what Freud says, and that he later abandoned the seduction theory. Then—and this is the important part—she says it wasn't my fault, which is shocking, because I always thought it must be.

'It is not your fault,' she repeats. 'It is not your fault.'

'I never want to talk about this again,' I say.

A week after this, Dr Finch sticks her head into the waiting room, and I glance up from a book I haven't been reading (looking at a book is a good way to look like you are doing something productive, as long as you flick your eyes about a bit and turn the pages from time to time).

She is five minutes late, which is nothing in the scale of a week. If I had to describe her in one word, I would say consistent.

We walk along carpeted corridors, then the stairs and the corridor to her office. I sit in my seat and wait for her to ask me how I have been. In a few seconds I will start spreading my secrets across the table while the clock ticks by 60 minutes. We will probably overrun because she is nice like that, but still at some point all too soon it will be time to walk back down the corridor and leave.

'How have you been?'

This is what I want to say:

All week I have been drawing our chairs, remembering the red flick of 'engaged' that traps your smile in the door. Trying to reflect in the wall has been agonizing; shadows say nothing, except that things aren't hollow; it's all just silhouetted madness on indifferent plaster. But there you came again! Reliable like the cuckoo. You ushered me down passages, opened the door, and today I'll see myself in you.

This is what I say: 'All-rightish. Also, I never realised.'

'What did you never realise?'

'How white the walls in this room are. It's overpowering.'

'It's because it's sunny today. I would put pictures up to distract from their whiteness, but you know what people are like. They'll start thinking they have all sorts of symbolic meanings and that I'm trying to convey secret messages.'

She shrugs theatrically.

She smiles.

I smile back.

I wonder if she tells me this because she thinks I am different to the others. Perhaps she is trying to tell me I ought to be. A fly is buzzing in the room; sometimes it lands on her papers.

I suddenly stop looking at the fly and start listening very hard because she is telling me something about herself, which hardly ever happens. 'When I was little,' she says, 'I couldn't stop imagining I was in a tree, shooting everyone who passed by.'

How should I take this confession? I decide the thing to do is to look her in the eye and say the magic words:

'It's just a thought.'

She laughs, a real, genuine laugh. I feel warm and happy.

There is a chip on the baseboard behind her chair where a circle of paint has flaked off. I decide to name the little brown dent Lily and pretend it is me. That way I can be in her office even when I'm not.

I'm doing politics homework in my dorm during one of my free periods the next day when someone knocks on the door.

'Coming!' I call. 'One sec!'

I'm in my towel. I put my uniform on, open the door, and think I might pass out.

She's standing right there—in the corridor outside my dorm. I try to speak, but my tongue won't collaborate with my brain.

'What are you doing here?'

Dr Finch smiles. 'Come on,' she says, 'we're going on a day trip.'

'But I'm—wearing my school uniform.'

'It doesn't matter.' Her smile is getting wider. 'My car's outside. Let's go.'

So I go with her.

And then we are sweeping down lanes in her little red car and her windscreen wipers are swishing back and forth, back and forth, even though it's not raining.

I'm terrified but so, so happy. Has anyone named this emotion before? I would call it whizzing. That is what we are doing, though we are going so fast I can't be specific about details, and the sheep we pass start to look like fallen clouds.

'The sky is falling!' I say.

Dr Finch laughs. 'What are you on about?'

She glances at me quizzically for what feels like a long time, but is probably only two seconds.

'Keep your eyes on the road!' I scream, giggling but feeling like we might be quite close to The End.

'I mean we're going so fast, the sheep in the fields look like clouds.'

'Like clouds?' She's laughing again. 'Are we flying, then?' I can see her putting her foot down on the accelerator and realise we're going even faster. Her foot looks determined, angry even, like it has a mind of its own. I'm momentarily captivated by her shoes; brown, flat, and stubby with a bit of gold chain across the tongue. I think they must be her only pair. I've never seen her wear any other. Maybe they are her work shoes, though; perhaps she has others at home. Does that mean she's working now? Are we flying?

'Lily?'

'Yes?'

'Would you try if your friend wasn't looking?'

No reply. Haven't got one, don't want to give one. Faster, faster, hedgerows are great wobbling green waves, branches are arms whipping past like a crowd holding their hands out to touch a superstar, faster, the white painted lines on the road are sprawling vertebrae, faster, somewhere a protective film is being lifted and I am seeing the blue of the sky unfiltered for the first time, faster—and then—out of nowhere—a rabbit—

Dr Finch's reflexes kick in: brakes,

command to tyres: left, left,

We swerve

off the road

into a ditch

and everything is silent as death, apart from the rise and fall of our breath, which indicates we are both still by definition living. She drops her head slowly forward onto the steering wheel, her hair splaying out over it.

'Oh shit,' she says. I look back at the road. There is no squished rabbit. Lucky rabbit.

We are lucky too, because aside from being a bit shocked, neither of us is hurt, and the car is fine.

'We went a bit fast there, didn't we?' says Dr Finch, with a nervous laugh that veers close to a sob.

We sit for a few minutes, gathering ourselves, and then Dr Finch decides that we've calmed down for long enough. She revs the engine and slams hard on the accelerator.

After a few revs we are back on the road, but this time she remembers herself and only drives about 30 miles per hour over the limit. The trees and hedgerows still rush past in a slightly aggressive torrent, but now I can pick out little details like individual leaves and splashes of red berries.

We drive for another half hour before she pulls over sharply, and the car jerks to a halt.

'It's here,' she says, half falling out the car door in her excitement and not bothering to shut it behind her.

'But this is just a field.'

'Come on!'

She's jumping over the barbed wire, lifting up her long, flowy skirt with one hand so it doesn't snag, before breaking into a sprint.

'Come on!'

I climb over the wire and run after her.

When I catch up with her, I'm panting hard, but Dr Finch hasn't broken into a sweat. I throw myself facedown on the ground, breathing in its sweet grassy smell, trying to regulate my heart.

'It's here!' She's grinning.

'Haven't you worked it out?'

I nod.

'Well?'

'It's your tree.'

'Yep. I liked it better than all the others; I picked it because it looked sturdy. I wanted to make a tree house, but I couldn't work out how to do it. I used to live about a mile away. I could show you the house if you like.'

'I'm okay here.'

'Okay, then.'

'Why did you want to shoot people?'

'I don't know. I think they infuriated me.' She turns and looks at me, almost sternly. 'Can you keep another secret?' she asks.

'Yes.'

And then she gives me a hug,

and all the while I
am wondering whether she means it or
if after she will climb up the tree
and shoot me.

Somewhere, a door opens. I open my eyes, and find I'm still at school.

'Are you okay?' asks Ellie. 'You need to wake up. It's time for class.'

I peek out from under the covers. 'I'll be there.'

16

Those Who Love Me

It is best not to think about the car journey that never was.

Instead, I focus on the homework she set me for the week. Using the principle of graded exposure, I am trying to resist recording words, starting with those that occur around people I care about least.

People I care about least are the ones I am never going to see again: passersby, train passengers, shop assistants, etc. I still record my actions around them, but the idea of not remembering everything isn't as terrifying as when I know someone personally.

After them come people I know a little: people in my school I'm not friends with, and most teachers.

On the highest level are people I really care about: selected teachers, friends, and family.

At the very top of this pyramid is Dr Finch. It is critical to make sure my actions around her are perfect.

Before She left, She said not to get too stressed about what I did around Dr Finch. She told me She didn't like her and that she didn't matter. When I told Dr Finch this, she said the reason my friend didn't like her was because she threatened her existence.

Now that my friend has gone, I am free to care about Dr Finch as much as I want. She has replaced all my friends and stormed her way to the top of the letter charts. When I am with her, I want my actions to be so perfect, it is difficult to focus on what she is saying. I record everything.

The problem is, I can't tell her that.

How strange, though, when the person you are seeing to help you deal with an issue *becomes* the issue.

At our next session, I make it all the way up the stairs to her office, only generating one letter:

'Sorry to keep you **W**AITING,' she says. 'When did you get here?'

'Don't worry,' I say, 'I only got here 10 minutes ago.' But what if it was more like 11 or 12 minutes, and she checks with the receptionist and thinks I'm a liar?

A single letter is very manageable. So I am proud of myself, ecstatic even, when:

She opens the door and I approach the chair I usually sit on. I see there are two **B**LACK SPOTS on it. Perhaps she will only notice them after I leave and think that it is me who left them there?

I sit down in the chair, and it squeaks. Does it sound as if I have done a **F**ART?

She asks me how I am, and a fleck of **S**PIT comes out when I say the *S* of 'Sort of okay.' Does she notice? I realise I have been **S**TARING AT MY LAP to avoid looking her in the eye. If I do that too much, she might think I'm coming on to her, but staring into my lap probably looks rude and obnoxious. So then I try not to be rude and attempt to look her in the eye.

But as I do this, my gaze crosses the top of her **V**-NECK SWEATER. Will she think I am a pervert? Next my **S**TOMACH makes a burbling noise, and the room is so quiet she definitely heard, which is disgusting in itself. I **A**POLOGISE for the disgusting noise. She says 'Stop apologising for your stomach rumbling. It happens to everyone, it's a normal thing that all bodies do.' Is she trying to tell me that I am annoying for apologising? She changes the subject. She asks me to draw one of my routines on a piece of PAPER. I do so and give it to her. But what if I didn't write down my routines, and instead I confessed to how much I love her, and she thinks I am weird and will never see me again?

WAITING, BLACK SPOTS, FART, SPIT, STARING, V-NECK, STOMACH, APOLOGISE, PAPER.

WBFSSVSAP.
WBFSSVSAP.
WBFSSVSAP.

I look at the clock. It hasn't even been five minutes.

'You seem distracted today,' says Dr Finch. 'I mean, you always seem a little far away, but today you're even further than usual.'

'Sorry. I really am sorry. My lists aren't so good. Sorry.'

'You apologise too much.'

'I know. It used to be a huge problem. I once won a prize for apologising . . . It was very embarrassing.'

'Can you think of someone who apologises the right amount and try to emulate them?'

'You,' I say. 'You don't apologise for no reason, but if you say something that's unfair, then you do.'

She shakes her head. 'The thing is, you really don't know me very well, so you can't use me as your model.'

Uh-oh, I think.

I do not know a single thing about the person who knows me best.

To love someone who is paid to be your friend is a terrible thing.

I am saying this to her. She stares back, doesn't say anything. Crosses and uncrosses her legs. Makes a note on her pad.

'Help me,' I am saying, 'please, please help me.'

I am no longer in my chair. I am curled up on the floor. I crawl across and wrap my arms round her legs. Dr Finch is very clever, and though when I first met her, I didn't think she was beautiful, I do now.

'I'm not going to let go, ever, I won't. Please help me.'

She chews her pen. 'I'm trying to.'

I fall asleep with my head on her lap while the clock ticks by an hour, and I wake up because she says quietly, 'That's all we've got time for now.'

I realise I've been in my chair all along.

I take my medication last thing before bed—an act of daily defiance towards my friend. I gulp them down guiltily. And not just because of what it does to her. Dad and Mum don't like me being on these pills. 'You have to think of Dr Finch like a priest,' says Dad. 'Medication is what her church, the psychiatric community, believes in, and so of course that is what she will preach. But that doesn't make it true. It's not necessarily right. I'm not convinced it's helping you. And I'm very concerned about the long-term effects.'

'It is helping me,' I squeak. But I can't deny that I've read the little folded leaflets that are slipped inconspicuously among the pills. They sit there in the packet, not causing any immediate concern, until you unfold them.

Dad goes on and on. He says I should do more sports, that endorphins and personal fitness are the answer. 'You are thin,' he says, 'but not fit.' I want to say, *I was at my fittest when my OCD was at its worst*. He says Dr Finch is toxic and wants to turn me against him. I don't know where he gets this idea from. I understand he had a phone call with her once. It did not go well. Dr Finch told me she had spoken to him. *Headstrong* was the word she used.

'There are specialists out there who would try to treat you without using medication,' he says. 'I could arrange an appointment for you with one. What do you think?'

No, I tell him, I only want to see Dr Finch.

'It seems to be very exclusive—this relationship between you and her. She's not telling me and your mum anything about what's going on.'

That's because, I should say, *I've asked her not to go into the details with you and Mum. I'm over 16. She won't tell you anything if I don't say she can. And I don't.*

At the moment my Bupa health-care plan is covering my treatment, but I don't know what will happen when that runs out.

Even though they are divorced, Mum agrees with Dad about the pills. She says she wishes I would give natural remedies and mindfulness a chance.

Mindfulness is the fucking problem: my mind is too full.
But I know my parents are being this way because they care. Because they want the best for me. Because they love me.

I have thought about this. Dr Finch thinks I should take the pills, but she will never love me. Mum and Dad don't want me to take the pills, and they will always love me. It is most important to keep close the people who love you unreservedly.

Therefore I will stop taking the pills.

'Dr Finch,' I say, 'I want to come off my medication. It's making my parents unhappy, and I can't do that to them. And I'm not going to come back for a while.'

She definitely has a response to this, but I can't quite work out what. Everything is coming out of her mouth in a rush; her jaw creaks and drops several inches to make a cave, spouting a rapid waterfall, foaming and gushing down her chest before soaking her trousers. She is staring at me with hollow eyes, saying everything and nothing at once.

But, I am thinking, she must be saying something. If I look closely, I can see that the cave is moving, annunciating, pronouncing, flashing between tunnels of teeth and tongue. Vowels and consonants and words are coming out. But what exactly? Everything she says seems silenced by the roar of falling water. At school I learned about sibilance. What is the intended effect of sibilance? This is something my English teacher once asked. I had to reply that I wasn't sure. I knew exactly how it worked, but I didn't know its point.

I feel the same now. I am absolutely certain that she is producing real sentences. I understand the mechanics, but I cannot see the point she is making. I briefly conjure up an image of her head on top of a printing press, hammering away with print all over her teeth.

What is the intended effect of sibilance?

'Do you have a strategy,' I hear, coming across the haze, 'if you are becoming more vulnerable to your routines while you're not seeing me, are you going to—'

And then on and on and more of that dreadful whooshing noise.

'Dr Finch, I don't care. You've told me before.'

She looks upset, but it's true. I didn't come here to be lectured. We've already been over everything I need to know. I came because I love her, because I want her to be my friend, and because she, the only acquaintance—is that the right word?—I have ever had who didn't want to tell me all about their life, is also the only person I ever wanted to know all about.

I end the session by saying I have to leave promptly, even though I have nowhere to go. (I worry about this lie all day, but it's better than being there a minute longer.)

'Okay,' she says, 'are you sure you don't want to go over anything else? Will you keep in contact while you are away? You know you can.'

I close my eyes and think about what to say next. I can hear her crossing the room, and I know she is behind my chair. She bends down, putting her arms round my shoulders, and I feel her hair float against my cheek, tickling like fleeting rays of sun in January. I open my eyes. She's sitting in her chair, looking at me over her papers, raising an eyebrow.

'Maybe,' I say.

We walk away from her office down the corridor, whose freshly painted smell I will surely drown in if the most important moments of your life really do flash past in your last living seconds. She looks at me.

'It feels like you're not coming back ever,' she says softly.

It is a thread of hope, and I cling to it. Is it possible that she is going to miss me?

'Good-bye, then,' she says.

I head out to my taxi. The driver stubs his cigarette out with an orthopedic-looking shoe, grunts, nods. 'Bye,' I say, without looking back.

There is going to have to be a grieving period. Without her, everything is dark. It is like her room in reverse.

And how exactly do my eyes see people?

She is everywhere. She is the backs of long skinny women who look willowy and slightly malnourished. She is the woman across the park sitting on the bench with her hair flying out behind her like telltales on sails. She is every person with fair hair, every person with blue-grey eyes, every person who is too hard-line liberal to wear makeup, and every person who has ever thrown me a sympathetic look. I cross streets to be closer to these people. I want to say something to them, but I have no idea what wouldn't sound completely weird.

This evening I see her face in the dips and swells of a cloud, so I climb up onto the roof of the house to be closer to it.

Now I am lying in bed with a fever.

How exactly did I get down from the roof? At the end of my bed I see a giant black Wellington boot, tapping up and down. There are words printed on hundreds of paper ribbons swirling out of it like steam from a cauldron. I try to catch them, and they dart back into the boot. They are so quick, they remind me of shoals of fish that appear composed until you try to touch them. I think they are teasing me. But I am resolute; I will catch one of them. I do catch one, but it disintegrates and ash falls through my sieving fingers back into the boot. But the words have been left behind and are hanging in the air, superimposed on the haze. They shimmer in black, fresh wet print, and I read them.

WE ARE LIVING IN AN AGE OF COPY AND PASTE.

Now that I have heard these words, I cannot forget them. I wish I hadn't seen them. I lie down again, but the room is spinning and the words are there and they will not go. The phrase will not leave me alone.

We are living in an age of copy and paste we are living in an age of copy and paste we are living in an age of

17

Thailand

I turn 18. School ends, and I defer my place at Trinity College, Dublin, for a year so that I can go travelling. To pay for it, I have worked in a nursery for a term, cleaning mouths, wiping hands, and finger painting. I have spent a lot of time taking pictures of children, because we have to photograph them for their progress files so that inspectors from the fascist Ofsted children's services can check them any time:

> This is Timmy washing his hands by himself for the first time!
> Below—Timmy engages in group play with his friends Ben and Jack. They are pretending to be bankers!
> Above—Timmy puts his thumb in clay to make a Divali candle. We are learning about other cultures!

Last week, I put the nursery's digital camera in the pocket of my smock so I could help kids wash paint off their hands without getting it wet. I accidentally forgot about the camera, and only remembered it when I got home and took my smock off. For child protection reasons, removing a camera from the nursery is an absolute no-no. Yet there I was, standing in my kitchen with the incriminating object.

I didn't sleep that night. At about 5.30am I threw up, in anticipation of the impending legal action by the nursery.

I considered throwing the camera in a skip and catching a taxi to the airport, but running always looks suspicious, so I turned up to work as normal, and everything was as it should be. The other teachers and assistants were milling around, setting up easels for the day and covering tables in newspaper. I carefully put the camera back in its drawer. By midday, when no one had said anything and everyone was still acting normal, I dared to believe that they hadn't noticed.

'Did the camera situation become a major problem in real life or just in your head?' Dr Finch would say if she were here. 'Do you think perhaps you should consider upping your meds again?'

No, I do not.

I have been coming off them sensibly and gradually for the last few months. I am one dose away from being off them for good. Yes, my lists are getting worse, but maybe travelling will solve everything; maybe I can fight this on my own. Mum and Dad traveled, when they were my age. They both talk about it like those were the best days of their lives.

'I know it hasn't been easy for you lately,' Dad said, when I told him where I planned to go. 'But I think it will do you the world of good—to get out there and do something like this.'

I am volunteering at an orphanage in Thailand. I will take two weeks of pills with me. When I have finished them, my withdrawal from medication will be complete.

Ella is 13 now, and she's just finished her first term at boarding school. She refused to go to Hambledon. 'Uh,' she said. 'I don't

want all the teachers there comparing me to 'perfect Lily.' And
I want to go somewhere with boys!'

The change in her was rapid. She went away with puppy fat
and frizzy hair—she came home for the holidays taller, slimmer,
with glossed lips and an iPod full of indie music.

I'm focusing on packing my bag while she flits around my
room, but then she starts to say something that demands my full
and complete attention:

'Lils,' she starts. 'I keep doing this really weird thing.'

'What?' I ask her. 'What do you do?'

'I . . . I . . .' She stops, sighs. 'No, I can't say. It's going to
sound too weird.'

'Tell me.' I beg myself to keep my voice level. 'Whatever it
is, I promise I won't say you're weird.'

'Okay.' She delivers her confession over my head, to the
ceiling. 'I feel like I have to hold my breath for a certain amount
of time, otherwise Mum will die. It started off as 10 seconds,
but it keeps getting longer, and now I'm doing it all the time.
It's horrible. I do it until my lungs hurt and my chest feels like
it's going to burst.'

It's bad enough that I live the way I do, but the idea of poor
little Ella being stalked by horrible thoughts is almost too much
to bear. I must be calm. I must not make her worried. What
would Dr Finch say? Think, think.

'That's a magical thought,' I say slowly. 'It's where you
mistakenly believe that something you do can cause or change
an unrelated event. They're quite common.'

'So I'm not really odd?!'

'No, you're not odd at all. The thing to do is not respond—
treat it as random background brain noise. You don't really have
any control at all over Mum's life. But the more you obey the

magical thought and hold your breath, the more the thought will come back and make you miserable. I know it seems hard, but next time you have the thought, don't hold your breath. Ignoring it the first time will make you really stressed. After a while, though, the worry you feel about ignoring it will go down, and if you don't engage with it, the thought will stop coming. Do you think you could do that?'

'Okay,' says Ella, nodding. 'I'll try. How do you know so much about this?'

I could tell her. I know I could trust her. Then I see her face, more teenage by the day, but still so young. So damageable.

'It's just something I find interesting,' I say.

'I'll miss you when you're gone,' she says.

'I'll miss you more.'

Pim, one of the carers at the orphanage, collects me from Phuket Airport in a pickup truck. Pim is gigantic and round, with kind eyes and a flat, sweaty nose. He wears a hot pink T-shirt that looks like it could double up as a tent. We leave the centre of Phuket and speed along a dirt road, Pim singing all the way— because apparently he will soon be a famous Thai rock star.

When we arrive, we are in a sandy courtyard with huts coming off it. Pim deposits my bag in my hut and flicks a lizard off the wrought-iron bed and out of the door. I see a ginger paw coming out from underneath the bed. I peek down to have a look, and a three-legged cat peeks back. 'Please refresh and take a look around,' Pim tells me.

The children are not back from school yet, and won't be for a few hours. The other huts are the same size but have no beds, just lots of dirty mattresses strewn across the floor. Have they given me their only bed? Am I the only one with my own room?

ONLY BED AND OWN ROOM is added to my list.

I'm supposed to be resisting making lists so that travelling can heal me, but I want to have a clear head when the children arrive. So I decide to go through what's happened so far and disregard the whole no-lists thing. Just one more routine: this is the last one, truly.

I hear a car pull in, and the courtyard echoes with voices. Children rush into my hut. The three-legged cat jumps out from under the bed and out of the window.

'Pee Antan!' they are squealing. 'Pee Antan!'

I vaguely remember Pim saying something about me getting a new name that means 'Sister Flower.'

They gather round me, pulling at my clothes, my arms, anything they can get hold of. One of them has jumped on the bed so she can be taller than me and is braiding my hair.

They are all talking to me so fast I can't make out individual sounds. I'd learned some key phrases from a Learn to Speak Thai book, but they disappear just as I need them.

So instead I parrot the noises they make. They find this so hilarious that they don't mind me not understanding them. They line up, pointing to themselves and trying to say their names louder than everyone else: Mook, Um, Cindy, Sea, Ka, Fah, Pupe, Ocean, Sun, Ali, Bim, Boom . . .

Dinner is served from an open-air counter by a friendly but tired-looking woman called Kamon. Flies land on the rice and curry, rubbing their front legs together.

I looked around the kitchen earlier. The surfaces were clean to the eye, but I've yet to see any cleaning products. Kamon probably washed her hands before cooking, but the soap is one of those suspicious white bars with brown in the cracks.

I take the portion ladled onto my metal tray and sit down in the courtyard with identical twins Bim and Boom. Pushing my food round, I decide that I can fall short-term sick. I'll have to cope with all the normal implications like vomiting and worrying I've been disgusting, but that's manageable. The problem is more if I get long-term sick:

Humans catch tapeworms by swallowing food or water containing traces of contaminated faeces.

'You no like?' says 11-year-old Pupe, who speaks the best English of the group and has already asked me to teach her new words. 'Eat up!'

I juggle whether I am going to feel worse if I cause cultural offense by saying I don't want to, or if I go along with it and worry later that I've caught an awful tropical disease.

I manage a few mouthfuls. Pupe smiles.

When Pupe, Bim, and Boom are finished, they pick up their trays and take them around to the back of the kitchen, where there's a large bowl of water that was probably once warm and soapy but is now lukewarm and brown from food. Rice, tomato, and chicken float in it. The curry sauce clumps at the surface, leaving an oily slick.

They dunk their cutlery and bowls, lift them out, shake them, and place them on the side. That's it. Washing done. They indicate that I should do the same.

She cackles: *Are you going to get sick? Or are you just a horrified little Western girl? What's worse?*

Oh! Her voice catches me unawares; it makes me think I

might drop my tray. I grip the tray so hard my thumbnails turn a strong pinky colour from the blood pumping beneath them.

It's been months since I heard from her.

Funny, the weeks I spent longing to hear that voice, and now that I have, I am filled with fear.

Go away, I say.

Nothing.

I shiver in the 40°C heat.

After dinner, I'm playing football with about 20 boys and girls when Pim pulls me to one side.

'It's nine. Shower time. Older ones do themselves. You wash younger children. Don't forget wash privates.' Pim laughs, groping his crotch to indicate the area of interest and making a lathering action. ' 'Shower' in Thai is *abnam*.' Then he wanders off.

I stand on the sidelines, panic mounting. How would you define young? What if I end up washing one of them who is actually capable of washing himself? Then it will look like I was just washing him unnecessarily for my own pleasure. Am I really supposed to scrub their privates—isn't the clue in the name?

'Abnam!' I call, hoping they don't notice that my voice is shaking. The older-looking children run off to their huts, so I'll assume they are the 'capable washers.'

The remaining children form a queue outside the shower room. They look at me expectantly.

The first one in the line, Cindy, flings off her T-shirt and trousers, skips into the shower room, takes a yellow sponge from the side, and dips it in a large bucket of water before handing it to me. She looks up at me expectantly.

I say to myself:

In the end it is all done.
In the end it is all done.
In the end it is all done.

I am sitting cross-legged on my bed, worrying I have hepatitis because I just scratched a mosquito bite and it's started to bleed.

Six-year-old Sea, the youngest in the orphanage, bursts into my room. She is in her pyjamas and clutching a blanket.

'Tonight sleep here,' she says, pointing to my bed.

I laugh nervously. Michael Jackson crashes into my thoughts; I cannot have children sleeping in my bed.

I can hear Pim talking to Fah in the courtyard.

'Pim!' I call. 'Pim!'

He pokes his head round my door.

'Pee Antan?'

'Yeah, Pim, could you tell Sea that she isn't allowed to sleep in my bed?'

'Why she no allowed sleep your bed?'

'Well, don't you think that would be a bit, er, unprofessional?'

'Why you say this word 'unprofessional'?'

'Could you just tell her she's not allowed?'

'Why she no allowed?'

Oh Jesus.

'I just, um . . . In England . . . um . . .'

Pim looks at me expectantly. Is he really that innocent?

'I no see problem.' He shrugs and wanders off.

And that's how I end up trying to go to sleep with a six-year-old curled up round me, playing with my hair and whispering 'Pee Antan?' in my ear every two seconds. I am trying to stay calm, but I worry this is all some sort of sick test.

What if OCD doesn't exist? What if after I told Dr Finch that I obsessively fear that people might think I'm a pervert, she actually reported me to the police? Imagine if all this—the showers, kids holding my hands, Sea getting into my bed—is a test and I am being filmed and the evidence will be used in court when I get home.

But how could it be a setup, when I decided to come here of my own accord?

Unless I was brainwashed?

I lie awake for hours, and before I know it, Sea is tickling my feet, calling for 'brek brek.'

When the children go to school, the orphanage takes on a bizarre still quality. I stay behind and wash the school uniforms in one of those open-topped 1920s bucket washing machines.

Ali, who was dumped at the orphanage last week by someone who sped off into the distance on a motorbike, helps me. Ali has never been to school. The local school won't take him until he meets certain standards. My job for the next few weeks while the kids are at school is to start teaching him. At the moment, he's 12 but can't even count to 10.

I'm checking the clothes carefully before I hang them on the washing line in the courtyard. I'm not sure exactly what I'm looking for, but I have a feeling I may have let some of the sterile needles from my first-aid kit fall into the washing machine.

Dr Finch has explained 'cognitive dissonance': where a person holds two contrary beliefs, such as 'I know I have not taken out my needles' and 'My needles might be in with the clothes.'

Giving it a nice little label doesn't make it any less terrifying. I run my hands carefully over a tiny faded orange T-shirt, and Ali tips his head at me. He is probably wondering what the hell

I am doing. I don't want to freak him out, so I try hard to stop feeling everyone's clothes.

When we're done, we make our way to the little table in the middle of the courtyard, and I lay out counters, dice, and some numbered cards. Pim wanders over and tells me I may 'be harsh, but not brutal.' When Ali refuses to sit down, Pim spins him upside down, pinches him on the bottom, and shoves his head into his armpit while counting to 10 in Thai. I can't imagine that Pim's armpit is a particularly nice place to be. I assume what Pim is trying to tell me is that I can basically discipline him however I like as long as he doesn't die.

Personally, I stick to my three-word Thai encouragement 'Yo yaan pe,' which means 'Don't give up.' It is quite effective until distraction kicks in, and he starts trying to eat the counters. Then he puts my stationery down his pants, and all I can think is that I am going to have DNA from Ali's genitals over my pencils. If that doesn't get me arrested, I don't know what will.

The children return from school, and we start weeding a plot of land that is going to become a vegetable patch. The orphanage wants to grow some of its own food and be more financially independent. Alas, these are no garden weeds; these weeds rise above your waist and have roots attached to clumps of wet mud the size of human heads. Huge spiders and fat slugs tumble down and land on your feet.

We do this for two hours. I'm in a bikini; the children have stripped down to their underwear. The mud has dried all over our bodies so we all look the same colour.

Not that I am looking at their bodies. I am not looking at their bodies.

Afterwards I join the children in the river that runs by the orphanage, washing and cooling down.

A mosquito bite on my leg has turned black and septic. If I push it gently with a finger, a green liquid oozes out. A redness is travelling up my leg, and I have hours to live. I should never have gone in the river.

'If you ever have a cut that looks infected, and you start seeing red lines going in the direction of your heart,' said Mrs Nelson in biology, 'you need to get medical assistance immediately. You probably have serious blood poisoning, which can be FATAL.'

I show Pim, who nods solemnly and confirms my worst fears: 'Must go doctor.'

Pim disappears, and a few minutes later I hear an engine revving and horn beeping from the road. Pim is sitting on a motorbike, patting the back of a torn leather seat and indicating I should get on.

It's difficult to put into words quite how much I do not want to get on a motorbike with Pim.

Equally, I do not want to die of septicaemia.

Pim grabs my arms and places them round his belly. His damp shirt clings to my arms. We set off down the dirt track in the direction I came from all those weeks ago. The wind whips my body—I'd forgotten what it is to feel cool. Goose bumps break out on my bare arms. What if Pim thinks I am sexually aroused because I have my arms around him?

Will he add this to the list of my sexual misdemeanours he will be reporting back to whoever organised this sick game?

We travel for around 30 minutes before we skid to a halt outside a little house.

Inside, Pim translates for the doctor, a small man in a stained white coat. Apparently, the whole of the infected bite must be removed, which will involve taking a small chunk of my leg out using a scalpel. It is important we do this soon, as the infection is spreading up my leg. The doctor will inject me with anaesthesia so I don't feel a thing.

This is the choice before me: die from the bite itself or die from catching a disease in the dirty operation. Do you remember the girl who went to Thailand and contracted HIV from the needle giving her a tattoo?

I do.

I brought clean needles with me in my first-aid kit that I could get out and use, but somehow they feel dirty just by being here. I turn down the anaesthesia. The doctor protests, shaking his head and waving his hands back and forth.

'It's going really hurt,' translates Pim. 'The doctor is no sure even strong man could take pain.'

But I am resolute. A scalpel is bad enough; it is my limit; it is as far as I can go. No needle will touch my veins. I have a small unused scalpel in the first-aid kit. I tell Pim to get the doctor to wash his hands in front of me. The doctor does as instructed, and I take the scalpel out of its sterile packet and pass it to him with shaky hands.

I lie back on the doctor's bed.

'Just do it,' I say.

Today is Saturday, and we are at a fair in the neighbouring town.

In England, large outings with kids involve meeting points, emergency procedures, and risk assessments. Here, Pim and Kamon wander off to buy food for the evening, calling over their shoulders, 'Pee Antan, watch children!'

I want to shout, *When and where shall we meet? And are any of them allergic to peanuts or carrying EpiPens?*

Before I can say any of this, at least eight of the 20 kids in my care shoot off into the bustling crowds. Shit. If they get abducted, is it my fault?

I urgently need to make some lists about how letting some of the children run off was irresponsible, but if I focus on that, I might lose even more.

'No worry!' says Bim, looking at my face. 'No worry!'

She takes me by the hand

(**H**AND HOLDING: A young girl held my hand, and I didn't try to stop it happening.)

and leads me to the pick-and-mix stall.

Mook, Cindy, Bim, Boom, and Fah fill brown paper bags from rows and rows of candied maggots, caramelised spiders, and stag beetles on sticks. They try to get me to eat a sugared locust. Would I rather cause cultural offense or have a dirty mouth? It's an easy one by now. Locusts every time.

'Open mouth!' says Boom.

I stick my tongue out, and Cindy plops it on my tongue.

I feel its sugary body fizz and disintegrate on my tongue, its legs crunching against my teeth.

'Good?' says Bim 'Good?'

Cause cultural offense or tell a lie? A lie every time.

'Delicious!'

Somehow, after an hour or so, chance upon the rest of them at the bumper cars. The fair is huge; it seems incredibly lucky. Perhaps I didn't do anything irresponsible. Perhaps there was just a larger plan I didn't know about. Then Kamon and Pim appear.

Pim counts the children and pats me on the back. 'Good job,

Pee Antan! Good job!'

My time in Thailand comes to an end, and on the way to the airport, I sit and wonder how long it is going to take for my body to shut down because of the ways I have contaminated myself here.

Sea, Bim, Boom, Mook, Pupe, and Ali wanted to come and say good-bye, so they're in the back of the pickup truck with me.

I see myself splashed across the headlines of newspapers in the Heathrow WHSmith bookshop upon my return, doomed to be forever archived among the bald 50-year-old men with clear aviator glasses who seem to make up the majority of the paedophile population. I imagine what it will be like when they lead me away in handcuffs and strangers spit at me.

On the positive side, Ali has mastered his ABCs, counting to 100, and a collection of vaguely useful English words. He has been accepted by the local school.

The journey takes about two hours.

The children hug me, and for the first time I feel relaxed, because hugging people you have known for a while when you leave them is a social protocol.

I cannot be accused of doing anything wrong.

After a few minutes of good-byes, the children climb into the back of the truck, and Pim shakes my hand before slamming the door. Then they start to drive away. Little Sea is wailing, and Bim is hugging her. I hear Pupe call 'H-A-M-B-U-R-G-E-R— HAMBURGER!' and 'G-O-O-D-B-Y-E—GOOD-BYE!'

They are waving and getting smaller and smaller. I watch until I can't see them anymore. I wonder how helpful it is for a child living in a remote Thai village to be able to order a hamburger in English. Then I take the sanitiser out my backpack so I can kill the bacteria from Pim's handshake.

When I arrive back at Heathrow, I am surprised there is no blue siren squad waiting to read me my rights. Only Mum and her fiancé Oliver, cheering at arrivals, saying how well I look.

18

Dublin

I'll leave for Dublin next week, and Ella, who has been home for summer, will be going back to school shortly after that. Already the days are getting shorter. We walk Tuffy in the park together in the afternoons, taking the dusty bridleway to the big lake looped by spindly trees, their shadows clawing across our path.

'Hey,' I ask, trying to sound offhand. 'You know the thoughts you were getting about holding your breath to keep Mum alive? How are they now?'

'They're good,' says Ella. 'I just did what you said, and they went away. I feel a lot better about the whole thing now.'

I am stunned. How come I can't do what Dr Finch tells me, but when Ella hears it second-hand from me, she gets it right away?

'That's amazing! Great. I'm so pleased.'

If she's fine, if she's *not* like me after all, maybe I can tell her. Not everything. But something?

'I'm thinking . . . I'm thinking that I want to tell you how I knew what you should do. The thing is, I have OCD. But not what you think of as OCD. I didn't realise I had it for a long time, because it's mostly in my head. The main thing I do is make lists of bad things I've done. But I've also had magical thoughts, which can be part of OCD. I've had thoughts about being able to control whether people I love get hurt, often you, in fact. I've seen a psychiatrist about it, and I'm trying to get better.'

'No way!' she says. 'I thought you knew how to tell me what to do because you're clever. I can't believe you didn't tell me! Tuffy, that is *not* your picnic!' Tuffy is 10 now, and selectively deaf.

'Well, I've told you now.'

I decide to go back on medication to make the thoughts go away. I'm on the lookout for my friend, wondering when She will jump out from behind the doorway of some dark thought.

Surprise! Happy failure to you! She'll shout, tooting a party horn with relish. *That's a nice little chemical dependency you've got going there. Harder than you thought without me, is it?*

Or perhaps She won't be so gleeful. She always hated the pills, after all; the way they dulled her shine. Maybe She'll swoop in and tell me not to take them—say that we could start over instead. But there's nothing, not a peep.

Taking the pills again means seeing Dr Finch a few times. There is a tension between us. We walk the corridors in silence, and talk in her office is purely strategic.

I am about to go to college and things will be fine. I'm not going to do my routines. This will be a fresh start.

'How?' asks Dr Finch.

'It just is. I'm going to a different country and starting again.'

'Then why didn't that work when you went to Thailand? We've only just got you stabilised on your meds again. We want things to continue getting better for you, don't we? I think you should think carefully about this.'

'That was different,' I tell her. 'I wasn't approaching things with the right attitude. I wasn't implementing all the CBT we've done in the right way.'

She raises an eyebrow.

I don't care.

I have finessed my system and its efficiency has been increased. There are now nine categories, and any bad action will fall into one of them.

This means I no longer end up with lists hundreds of letters long. Also, I now write down my bad actions rather than storing them in my head. This is sound, as it means I cannot lose any. Because someone might find my lists if I use a notebook, I've chosen to type them out in the notes section of my securely passcoded iPhone. When I get to the end of a routine, I still do my moving actions to close it and repeat my mottoes. Then I get Blank Slate, as before, and the whole thing starts again when I next do something wrong.

The categories are:

BODILY FUNCTIONS
LIAR
BORING/ LOSER
PERVERT
IDIOT
BITCH/ UNKIND
RUDE
POSH TWAT/ SPOILED
SELFISH

Trinity College's Halls are located in Dartry Road, Rathmines, a 15-minute drive from the centre of Dublin. Foreign students are bussed there from the airport, in nervous silence. Instinctively, I add **A**WKWARD to my list as penance for not mustering up an engaging conversation. I put it into the category *LOSER*, before mentally slapping myself.

Resist.
Resist.
Resist.

I am assigned to Cunningham House, the oldest hall on the block. In its entrance hall, I meet a girl called Aoife, who says I should feel free to 'come visit' her on the third floor and 'hang' any time I like. Just being in the presence of a future proper friend sends me into overdrive.

OVERKEEN, **S**TARED AT HER BOOBS, and **BR**EATH SMELL spring up like unwanted weeds, and though I smile on the outside, my stomach starts to twist.

Once I've shaken off Aoife, I locate my room at the end of a corridor on the second floor. I lock the door, and my suitcases fall from my clenched fists. I lie on the bed and order the words that have popped up into their appropriate categories, rapidly hammering them into my phone.

The kitchen is about 10 metres from my room, but paper-thin walls mean I can hear voices and laughter from the corridor. My new friends have arrived. I walk towards the babble, without generating a new word. I push open the peeling orange door and the conversation stops. Six expectant heads turn my way. The room smells of pizza and feet.

'Hi! I'm Lily!' I grin, feeling like an *IDIOT*. Smiles all round.

'Pull up a chair!' says a tall, waif-thin girl with long red hair. Keela.

'Where are you from? Not Ireland, I guess?' This question comes from a girl twirling a strand of her hair around her finger at the other end of the table.

'Haha! You got me. I'm from London.'

What kind of *POSH TWAT* says 'You got me'?

'Oooooh. London!' they chorus.

I smile in what I hope is an appropriate way, take a seat on a devastatingly squeaky plastic chair—please don't let them think I am farting—and try not to do anything seriously wrong.

This works well until my general tepidness causes a torrent of words to spin into the *BORING* category. Perhaps I should lead the conversation and impart wit and charm? Perhaps I should host the gathering, and, at the cost of generating hundreds of words for the list, shine bright?

I try it.

Freshers Week dawns grey and drizzly. So far I've acquired four main friends: Molly, Deirdre, Nessa, and Keela. Cunningham is a single-sex accommodation, but the boys' compound is linked to ours. Integration of the sexes is going to be crucial to successful first-year life, so we're relieved that the boys waste no time infiltrating our kitchen on night one. We rally ourselves with drinking games where the numbers and characters on playing cards take on strange meanings. *King—make a rule! Nine—bust a rhyme! Six is dicks! Drink up lads! Jack—never have I ever . . .*

Throughout the day, I've teetered between making sure I'm not boring and disappearing to write down generated words. Currently I can't keep up with the speed of words being produced, so I just type down the word and promise myself I'll do a full report of the content later.

I check the time: 8pm. I'm frazzled. In front of me, a bottle of vodka and a plastic cup beckons. *Four is whores! Drink up girls!* Yippee! I tip my head up to the ceiling and drink.

Music pumps. Lights flash. I love these people. These people are my friends. They love me back. I am accepted. These people. Are so beautiful. I smell of vodka, but I am free. I took some pills, and I am flying. Genuinely—there are wings fluttering in my stomach. This is it. Right here. In this nightclub. We were dancing and I bumped against Molly's bum but it doesn't matter. I am not a pervert because it was an accident. She knew that. I knew that. This is me. This is life!

In the morning, my head is over the toilet, retching. I woke up after two hours with a stomach full of vomit. It's now midday, and things haven't let up. I'm not the only one. Chunks of sick lined the toilet bowl before I even contributed. If other people are sick, does it cancel out my disgustingness?

Getting so drunk my memory fails results in Blank Time. But there are troublesome implications. Endless possibilities that I can't account for. Did I tell lies compulsively? Did I shit myself on the dance floor? Perhaps I sprayed a fleck of saliva on someone during a drunken conversation?

E-mail to Dr Finch:

Hi, Dr Finch,

I am sharing a bathroom and kitchen with seven other girls, and encountering the same problems I experienced when living with a group of people at school. I am constantly scared that I have left fingerprint smudges and skin cells behind, or something in the kitchen sink or on the floor. I keep checking everywhere, though I'm really not sure what it is I have left behind. I found a piece of fluff in the kitchen cupboard that was the same colour as the wool on my sweater. I thought, thank god I checked so that I could find the fluff and throw it in the bin, that was a close call, but fluff isn't really incriminating so I think I must be looking for something else.

I am also stressed that the people I live with think I am doing very bad things, but that's just usual so not much to be done I think.

Hope you are well,

Lily

Dr Finch asks, What would really be so bad about leaving evidence of your presence behind? Everyone else does it and is not concerned by it. Tackling OCD involves taking risks to find out what actually happens and whether or not it is as bad as feared.

She signs off her e-mail 'Rachel.'

After a few days, my reputation precedes me. I'm a legend, mostly known for things that happened during Blank Time—things I don't remember.

'Have you met my English friend Lily? She's crazy fun. Like properly nuts. You should hear what she did last night.'

This is my standard introduction. God knows what they say about me behind my back.

The only category I have conquered is *BORING*. Everything else is worse. All time not partying is dedicated to routines. I get about two hours' sleep a night; often I don't go to bed at all. There isn't enough time.

Diet Coke is my weapon.

Which is not to say I don't get into bed: I spend hours there every day. People don't disturb you if they think you are asleep, prompting less human contact and fewer routines. Lying as still as possible reduces words too.

I've begun to think there are cameras in my room. These days, even scratching an itch on my arm in private needs to be written down in *BODILY FUNCTIONS*.

If someone does come into my room, I'm desperate for them to leave as soon as possible, because I've started to worry that the room smells bad. Personally, I can't smell anything, but that doesn't mean there isn't a bad smell. I spend hours sniffing my sheets, clothes, books, and folders, searching for smelly traces and inspecting for fingerprints and old skin. I'm worried that it is my actual body that stinks, but, inconveniently, I have to take myself everywhere.

Showering and toileting are a mission. I've decided to stop eating most of the time, because it means I won't have to poo in the communal toilet. A benefit of avoiding food is that I don't risk poisoning myself or others, and that I won't leave fingerprints or traces of skin in the sink, fridge, cooker, or anywhere else unsanitary. When I can no longer ward off the hunger pangs, I have a bowl of Ready Brek cereal. In the terrible event that I have to defecate, I go to McDonald's drenched in shame and pray I don't see anyone I know.

It's easier to pee in the sink in my room and disinfect the area afterwards. I take responsibility for all hair and anything else (skin, nails, you name it) in the shower the seven of us share. Every time I shower, a new wave of communal body debris has arrived, which I pick out and discard, so no one can think it's mine.

I've become a compulsive liar. If I tell someone I did something an hour ago, but actually it was an hour and six minutes ago, I'm a liar. If I tell someone I'm going to my room to get something, but actually I'm escaping to do my routines, I'm a liar. If I tell Keela that Deirdre had asked where she was, before remembering that Deirdre actually asked 'Have you seen Keela?,' I'm a liar.

The college has a student counselling service, so I ask if someone can help.

The counselling offices are around the corner from the main campus, just a few doors down from the National Art Gallery. On the appointed day I make my way towards the large rising block of glass that I recognise from the website. I hunch forward against the cold, my collar up and scarf wrapped around my neck three times.

Inside on the third floor, pastel-coloured furniture, plastic plants, and a cheery receptionist make me feel a little more positive. But then I spy a friend of Keela's in the waiting room. Oh, the shame, the burning shame. Her eyes flick up at me and then quickly down. Perhaps she feels the same?

My counsellor is a lady in her thirties, Gail, who has brunette mid-length hair. I have three appointments with her over the next few weeks, during which time she asks me about my childhood, my family, and my life now. What do I find stressful about college?

She *mmm*s a lot. She says 'Uh-huh,' 'Why's that?' and 'How did that make you feel?' Her specialty is nodding.

I answer her questions, and she doesn't respond.

'Why don't you talk? You ask me, like, 10 questions a session, and the rest of the time you just nod and don't say anything.'

'That's how psychotherapy works. I'm trying to give you the physical space to verbalise your feelings, with no interruptions or time constraints. Silence isn't bad. This is a much-needed window of tranquillity for you.'

'Well, I don't mean to be rude. You're very nice. It's just . . . This isn't really helping me.'

'Mmm-hmm. What makes you say that?'

College is a 30-minute cycle from the dorm, so I purchase a bike in the hope that cycling will free me from routines.

Unfortunately, the bike is a useless therapist; Blank Slate will not come. Instead, getting on the bike means more time to review the day's words. This is how I come to be crossing a notoriously dangerous junction, muttering the categories:

LIAR
RUDE
SPOILED
BODILY FUNCTIONS
and
UNKIND

over and over under my breath. Around, me, traffic whizzes by in a whir of colour and noise that feels near but not near at the same time. I am fully in tune with the hum of my head, homing in on the points that make me *SPOILED*:

BOARDING SCHOOL: I told Molly I went to boarding school.
GAP YEAR: She asked me if I took a gap year, and I said yes.
FUNDING: She then asked me—whoosh!

A black four-wheel drive starts to turn left and hits my right side. I spin over the handlebars, landing splayed under the bike in a heap of torn jeans, grazes, and bike chain.

Cars swerve to avoid me with emergency screeches, horns blare, and a woman, who turns out to be the driver of the black car, screams. I sense the screaming may stop if I can demonstrate that I am alive. Am I alive?

Yes, I think so. Incredibly, nothing seems to hurt. Though I am lying still. Perhaps the pain will come if I move?

What categories should I sort this event into?

'It's okay.' I stand up, surveying the damage, which does appear to be only some holes in my jeans and multiple scrapes. 'I think I'm all right . . . It was my fault.'

'No, it bloody wasn't!' yells a man in a white van.

'The driver didn't signal!' says a man in a Corsa, who is so aggrieved he has parked his car on the pavement and is screaming at black-car woman.

'Genuinely, I think I'm fine,' I reply, trying to keep my voice level.

Black car woman is wailing.

'I've never done anything like that before,' she howls. 'I honestly don't know what happened. I'm so sorry.'

I try to evaluate the situation, which is difficult, as my half-finished routines are tugging at my sleeve like an annoying child in want of attention.

'I'm fine,' I manage.

I get back on the bike, pedalling furiously to the tutorial I'm now late for, beginning my routines from scratch and adding **A**TTENTION SEEKER to the category of *SELFISH* for causing such a scene. Later, when I see my bruised and cut body in the shower, it occurs to me that I was quite lucky.

This evening I am drunker than I've ever been. I call Dr Finch. She doesn't pick up. I text. I tell her that she clearly doesn't care.

I get the tram into town with friends. I drink more. I dance. I drink more and pass out. Someone takes me home. Crawl into bed.

When I wake up, it takes a couple of seconds to remember

what I've done.

Dr Finch. My phone. Shit.

I fumble on the bedside table. My phone's not turning on. I wobble across the room to jam it in the socket to charge. The screen stays black.

This phone has all my lists since I've arrived in Dublin saved on it. I haven't backed them up because I'm scared about replicating them. Hundreds of hours of meticulously crafted documentation of all the things I've done wrong in this academic year. Inaccessible. And I've been getting so drunk, I definitely can't remember them without it.

There is no way I can take it to be fixed, because what if the people at the phone place see my lists, pick out my worries about being a pervert, and call the police?

A vague memory of me throwing the phone at a wall when Dr Finch didn't reply takes shape . . .

Dr Finch!

I need to know what I said. If I know her at all, she will have replied by e-mail. Usually I hate her stuffy professionalism, but thank god for it now! I jab the power button on my laptop, waiting nervously as my e-mails kick into life.

One unread message. E-mail to Lily:

Hi Lily,

Me not picking up the phone is nothing to do with whether or not I care, but is about whether or not I'm in a position to talk. I always warn people that if they ring me outside office hours I can't guarantee to be available, and I'm sure you realise there are many possible reasons why that might be the case.

If you had left me a message the first time you rang, saying that you needed to speak to me urgently, then actually I almost certainly would have rung you back on that occasion. However, I had gone to bed by the time you sent the text telling me who you were.

I am sorry that you feel so negatively about your relationship with me. I did and still do genuinely care about you, and I think between us we did develop quite a good understanding of what was going on for you. Our relationship was different from friendship in some important ways, and these differences are what actually made it valuable, so meeting in another situation would have been very different.

You're clearly in a painful place at the moment, but I hope that, in time, you will be able to hold on to the positive aspects of the work we did together.

With best wishes,

Rachel

The e-mail is like a smack. I don't reply, as it would generate words and I don't have a phone to write them down on. Instead, I swig from the vodka in my top drawer and try to forget about it for a bit. Only when I am fully fired up with liquid courage do I type:

I don't want your best wishes, they stink. I don't think you have ever cared. I have been too upset because of you for too long and it must end. I know I have been unreasonable. Good-bye.

I have been arrested for stealing a handbag from under a table in a nightclub. I got caught because rather than bothering to leave, I carried on dancing with it.

Two burly officers push me into a cell and order me to strip to my pants, so they can be sure I don't have anything bad on me.

I don't have any money for bail, and I can't think who to call, so I stay in the cell overnight, reading the desperate messages people have carved on the walls (and wondering what they wrote them with if they had been properly strip-searched):

I only did it because I Love Jenny
Why the fuck won't they bring me any toilet paper? CUNTS
Please god anybody somebody help
Jo was not here
Facebook me;) Tim Lincoln #thisplacesucksass
Tracey likes black men's cocks

I start pulling out clumps of my hair. I don't know why. I suppose it is something to do. I pull more, until it's all over me and the floor.

An officer comes in. 'Stop doing that please,' he says. 'You're hurting yourself.'

I keep going, ripping at my scalp. Hair, hair, everywhere.

'Stop doing that please, you're hurting yourself.'

A few more hours later another officer comes in.

'All right,' he calls, 'time's up! You can go now.'

I don't move.

'I said you're free to go. Come and sign your release papers.'

I shake my head.

'Don't want to go home?'

'No.'

'Who's at home that you don't want to see?'

'No one.'

'Well, then, there's no reason to stay here. Besides, you can't. This isn't a hotel!'

He leads me down to the office, where tired-looking policemen and women with grey skin are chugging coffee. I look at the clock on the wall: 4.50am. A woman gets my stuff, which is in a little box with a sticky label on it, saying in felt-tip L. BAILEY.

I exit the police station and find myself squinting into the cold, walking in the direction of the river Liffey, where I use my last 10 euros to pay for a cab back to the dorm

'Long night?' asks the cabdriver, craning round and grinning at me with yellow, tar-stained teeth. My head is spinning with words, phrases, and categories, but there are so many, I don't know where to begin.

I try to focus on the facts.

I got so drunk, I decided that it was no use, all this trying to be good. So I did a bad thing to end all bad things, because scratching your nose or wondering if someone thought you were boring just don't seem so bad once you have broken the real and true law of the land.

But I got caught doing it.

And now, in the morning, my rebellion seems both pathetic and terrifying. The years I have spent trying to be good are dwarfed by this thing.

My lists are still gone.

Dr Finch does not love me.

Now I know what to do. I am admitting defeat. I have lost.

Previously when I toyed with the idea, the possibility, I had all sorts of vain ideas about how it might go.

I imagined I would listen to Pachelbel's Canon, because I always wanted that to be played when I walked down the aisle. And if I'm not going to get married, it will at least have an airing. I thought I might write letters to the people I loved, containing apologies and some sort of explanation. I pictured myself putting on my favourite outfit and doing my makeup with extra care, as if I were about to go somewhere important.

I planned to take my things in suitcases to the dump, because I couldn't bear the thought of everyone going through my stuff, trying too hard to understand.

I suppose I thought it would be a landmark event that I would need to prepare for. But now the time has come, it's not like this. It's just a normal December day, cloudy with a chance of rain, nothing special. The memories of my life will not montage themselves into a great black-and-white crescendo.

I am just tired, and I have had enough. My phone is still broken. I could continue to write my lists on paper, but it feels futile, knowing that I have lost so much vital content. It is like finding out your house has been burned to the ground, wandering round naked, lost, and cold, and then being told to build another house, despite having no money or resources.

My brain feels broken.

I write an apologetic note to Dr Finch so that she knows it isn't her fault, and put it in my desk drawer. Then I shower and shave my legs, because I don't want the coroner to think I am disgusting. I do several nervous pees, like a child about to embark on a long car journey with limited toilet access.

On the whole, I feel quite calm. It is as if I am about to write an unappealing essay that I've put off for a while but am now relieved to be finally getting on with, finding it easier than expected.

I put on my pyjamas. Then I take every pill in my bedroom and get under the covers, ready for the long sleep.

19

It Is My Fault

There is a man by my bed, his voice coming to me in waves.

Lily?

Can you hear me?

'Can you tell me how many pills you took?'

I can't.

I can't do anything.

I can't sit up.

Deirdre is in my room, along with lots of other people I don't know. 'Oh my god,' I can hear her saying, 'I should have checked on her earlier—it's just she often sleeps for a really long time—shit. I should have—shit.'

They must have called an ambulance. How long have I been in here for? A day? Two days? When did I go to sleep?

Can you tell me how many pills you took?

Pills.

Pills.

There are all kinds of popped blister packs around me in the bed. I am lying on some of them. I took so many. How am I awake again? This was not supposed to happen.

Can you tell me how many pills you took?

I try to make words come out. I—

don't—

know—
I am remembering.

Me: I don't believe in failed suicide attempts.
Dr Finch: Why not?
Me: I just don't. It's the sort of thing you have to get right first time round. Otherwise you obviously aren't completely sure.

I have failed. I couldn't even get this right.
Can you tell me where you are?
I—
I'm—
dark?

My body shakes like the aftershock of an earthquake rippling through every part of me. I feel myself palpate on the white sheets. A nurse swims into my line of vision, tightening something round my arm that goes *vvvvzzzrrr* and squeezes like too many people on the Tube. I try to tell her that a natural disaster is occurring inside me. She says that's the after-effects of the pills, and that it's my fault for taking so many of them.

It is my fault.

The thought rushes through me, chasing after everything like a wild wind in a carless tunnel on a very black and cold night.

It
is
all
my
fault.

Very high blood pressure, she says. I see the words jiggle in front of me and remember the letter magnets we had on the fridge when I was small.

V e   b l o o   s u r e
    r y h i g h   d p r e s

I'm not sure if she is talking to herself or me.

I' g o i n   g e t a   t o r
   m   g t o   d o c

She calls for someone, and the colour drains from everything until everyone around me looks like a sketch. A mad, bad picture. Knowing that any second now there will be—blackness again

20

Mental Ward

I've been transferred from intensive care to the psychiatric unit. It's a state place, and the rumours are true: it feels like a scrapyard for brains.

I'm in a room with four other people. The woman opposite me is screaming that the nurses are monsters and the doctors are devils pretending to be gods and even the orderlies are demons. Someone has given her flowers, but she has thrown them and now they are lying dead like soldiers on a linoleum battlefield.

Next to me is a nice middle-aged woman who keeps repeating the same things and forgetting what she said five minutes ago. She has asked me my age four times. Four times I have told her: 19. She can't stop dribbling; the front of her sweater is drenched. She tells me I am pretty over and over. She says I don't look crazy, and that I am too young to have troubles. She asks me if I have 'the anorexia.'

On the far side of the room is probably the ugliest woman I've ever seen. She is sweaty and vast, with wrinkles that look like they've been chiseled in by a drill. She has been staring at me and farting for the last half an hour. She sits on her bed in a hospital gown, with her legs crossed. She isn't wearing any underwear. A nurse keeps pulling down her gown and talking about 'modesty,' but it's no good, it just rises back up. I try not to see the thick bush and saggy pink folds of skin, but I already have done. I am a *PERVERT*.

I can't believe I'm not dead.

The most effective method would be to throw myself in front of a car or train, but I don't want to ruin someone else's life too. I need to jump off something, and make sure I don't land on anyone. I need to get to the top of the hospital. The windows may be locked, but that's okay. I can smash one. I get out of bed. I walk down the corridor to the end of the ward, where I encounter two security guards in front of a coded door.

'What do you think you're doing, girlie? This is a high-security ward. You don't just leave. Go back to your room.'

Deirdre and Nessa visit. They have brought me clothes, a wash bag, and a book.

'We brought you *Peter Pan*,' says Deirdre, handing me my tatty blue copy.

'I know it's your favourite.'

I flick through the pages, staring at the black-and-white illustrations I used to trace with my finger when I was small.

They are kind to me. They don't judge. They stay with me, sitting on the end of my bed. I am grateful they are here, but panicking—because words are arriving on my list thick and fast, and without a pen and paper to write them down, I feel stranded.

'You scared us, Lily. I mean, you really, really scared us,' Nessa says.

'We called your parents. We had to,' says Deirdre. 'They're on their way.'

The psychiatrist is about 50, with a grey mop of hair. He wears shabby brown trousers and a shabbier shirt.

We talk for half an hour. He seems friendly enough. He asks me what drove me to the edge. His voice is lilting, firm but soft at the same time.

'I'm a bad person. I spend my life trying to be good, and it's never enough.'

'Is there anything else?'

'I love my doctor. I'm obsessed by her. It's not an OCD thing. Actually, I think it is. Oh, I don't know anymore.'

It shocks me that I have said these words out loud. I want to undo them; Command Z the air.

'Mostly, I'm just a very, very bad person. I don't deserve to exist.'

'Do you know what I see?'

I shake my head.

'I see an intelligent girl who has a decision to make. Are you going to pick yourself up and do something with that intelligence, or are you going to throw it all away because right now, at this point in time, you don't feel like a good person? Anyway, I can't see anything bad. I mean, sure, you're English. But you can't help that now, can you?'

Dad arrives that evening; he got the first flight from London. He strides onto the ward purposefully with a big bottle of Lucozade.

Then he crumples onto the end of my bed. He sits and asks 'Why, why, why?'

'I don't know, I don't know, I don't know,' I say.

He tries to persuade me to eat the fizzy snakes and jelly sweets he bought at the airport.

I don't want them, but when he's gone, I eat them all.
I am ravenous.

Mum arrives the next day. She has flown in from Thailand, where she was doing a four-week yoga course that I didn't think about when I took the pills. She is tanned, but there's no glow. Her eyes are full of tears. She tells me she is so glad I am not dead. So, so glad.

They take me for lunch at the hospital café. This is the first time in forever I've seen my parents at peace. There is a weird sense of camaraderie. They say things that make me laugh; they tell me they still love me.

I'm trying to focus, which is difficult because for the last 24 hours I've been storing the lists in my head instead of writing them down.

They tell me it's time to go home. I thought I'd been sectioned, but they have persuaded the hospital that better treatment is available in the UK. While I was sleeping, Dad went to the police station and sorted out the mess, so I won't have to attend a court date. He also spoke to the college, and apparently I'm not going to be in any trouble. Mum is going to help me get my things. I am so very lucky that I have parents who love me as much as mine.

Back on the ward, the dribbling woman comes over to my bed, speaking quickly, her face nearly touching mine.

'If you're going home, luvvie, can you do me a favour? I have family and I'm not allowed out. But I'm sure they're going to visit me here this Christmas. Can you get them gifts? Anything you like; chocolate, perfume—the expensive stuff.' She presses 40 euros into my palm. 'Please? It would mean the world to me.'

I'm not sure what to do. Maybe this family isn't coming, and the presents will sit by her bed, making her feel worse. Maybe she really needs these 40 euros; maybe this is not the right thing to spend them on. I look at Mum. She is nodding obligingly. I'm too tired to make decisions.

Half an hour later, Mum and I are back with perfume and chocolates and 10 euros change. I give the woman a box of chocolates I bought for her myself, because although I really hope her family does exist, they might not, and I want her to have a present. She starts crying and telling me I am beautiful, and that she hasn't had a Christmas present in years. She is holding my hands in hers and asking why God has blessed her by allowing me into her life.

Then I tell her gently that I have to go. She nods.

'I understand, dearie,' she says. 'This place isn't for everyone.'

Mum and I get a taxi back to the dorm and start chucking things into bags at full speed, like looters: books, T-shirts, stationery, shoes, linen, towels, dresses, shampoo, posters. I take the unopened letter to Dr Finch out of the top drawer and place it carefully in my handbag. We haul everything into the hallway and lock the door.

Deirdre, Molly, and other girls from my corridor are hanging around outside, unsure of the appropriate etiquette to use.

'Apparently you had appendicitis,' says Molly. She looks hurt at being out of the loop. I know she knows. I piece things together. Deirdre and Nessa are the ones who know. Everyone else just *know knows*.

21

Harley Street

I've been home for a week, festering, writing endless lists. A notepad has become the new storage form. It has pros and cons, but I can't risk losing my lists again by putting them on a new phone. Mum and Dad say it is important that Ella is not told the full extent of what happened. She was at boarding school when I got back, so she doesn't know the circumstances of my arrival home. Mum lets her believe I'm just here for Christmas. She peeks into my room every couple of days, lingering uncertainly by the door and tugging her sweater sleeves down over her thumbs, asking if I want to 'do something.'

'No, no,' I say.

Yesterday she crawled into bed with me, nuzzling up to my side like she used to when we were small. Her skin touched mine; my flesh sizzled. I saw my hands at her breast, though I knew they were clamped by my sides.

'No, no!' I said.

'I don't get it,' she replied, lower lip wobbling. 'I was so excited about you coming back, but you don't want to see me. I feel like I've lost you.'

As for Mum, she has employed different approaches, and all in such rapid succession it's like watching a camera whiz through a day in one location in the space of 20 seconds. Blue sky that is obliterated by foamy clouds charging in from the left, pink seeping in from the corners of the frame tells you the sun is setting, a bird soars across like a rocket, nighttime—a spray of stars, dawn, then back to blue . . .

She was patient at first. She asked me if I wanted to talk; she suggested going outside for walks; she tried to understand. But I kept telling her not to come in please and that I wanted to be alone.

When I didn't change my tune, she became a stroppy teenager. She was textbook. I'd seen this act 1,000 times before from girls at Hambledon. 'Okay, fine.' She shrugged. 'I just don't think it's good for you to be in your room all day. But whatever.'

Passive enough on the outside, sure. But fire within.

On Wednesday it rained love. 'I love you so much, do you know how much I love you? Do you know that I would do anything in the world to make you better? And do you know how loved you are, by Ella, Dad, and Oliver too?'

But the love didn't fix me, so now, for the inevitable—

Mum stands at the end of my bed, the mug of tea that served as her excuse for entry slopping over the sides.

'So are you going to come downstairs at any point today?'

'No.'

'Are you going to do *anything* today?' She takes a step towards me.

'No. Please don't come any closer.'

'You can't do this!' She slams the tea down on my desk. 'You can't just . . . disappear! I mean, for god's sake, it's ridiculous! Pull yourself together!'

I must not shout.

'It's making everyone so unhappy. I'm at my wit's end. Poor Ella doesn't know what to think. But most of all, it's destroying *you*!'

I must not shout I must not shout I must not—

'We all want you to just be okay! *Why* are you being like this?'

'DO YOU THINK I WANT TO LIVE LIKE THIS? Do you think that I wake up in the morning and say, 'You know what would be really fun, let's spend hours and hours locked in my head, let's not leave my room, and hey, while we're at it, let's cut out all the people who care, because there really is nothing better, no, I cannot think of *anything* I would like to do more, than to reject the perfect, happy life I could have, and choose instead to live stuck on repeat in my own private hell'?'

'I just don't understand . . . why . . .'

'You don't understand? Well, that makes two of us. Why? You want to know why? *I* want to know why. Genetics? Upbringing? Just bad fucking luck? Guess what. I don't know, you don't know. All we get to know is that this is my life. And now'—I take what feels like my first breath in minutes, an ugly, shuddering gasp—'I would like you to leave.'

It happened.

I got angry. I sentence myself to weeks of remorse.

'Please,' I say. 'Just leave. I'm begging you.'

She makes to leave, but stops, hand wavering an inch above the door handle.

'All I want,' she says slowly, 'is for you to be open. You never tell me anything. I can't believe it got to this point and I had no idea how bad it was. I don't want you to have to deal with this on your own. I want to help you, but you need to let me in.'

It's been decided I should be assessed, so one Tuesday I end up in a waiting room on Harley Street. It's one of those posh waiting rooms that distinguishes itself from a National Health Service waiting room by having in-date magazines spread across the coffee table. And not just any in-date magazines: *Vogue* and *Tatler*. I suppose I should be thankful that if I have to go mad, at least I get to do it in a fashionable, aristocratic way.

When I look up from the coffee table, I notice a mahogany cabinet with some expensive-looking old books. *Darwin: The Beagle, Encyclopaedia of Tropical Diseases, The Complete Poetical Works of Robert Browning*, and *The Standard Edition of the Complete Psychological Works of Sigmund Freud*.

This would be all very cutting-edge if it were 1912, but I want to scream *It's 20-FUCKING-12!* I sit down on the button-back sofa. Why am I allowing myself to get so worked up about some old books? Is irrational anger a symptom of my condition? And while we're on the subject, what exactly is my condition? I'd quite like for someone to explain. What I experience is so unlike the OCD people have on TV.

Have they got it right?

In the corner there's a piano, in case some poor soul becomes so overwhelmed with the melancholic beauty of the situation that they feel the need to transmit their soul into sound. I'm tempted to go over and start hammering away the theme to *Jaws*.

The receptionist's smile is too big for her face. She says in a syrupy voice that it can't be very nice for us, sitting in silence: Wouldn't we like some music? My mother says yes, please. So the girl bends over, giving us a generous view of her pert pencil-skirted bottom, and turns on the radio. Smiling like she's done us a big favour, she sashays out of the room, clipboard under arm, off to rescue anyone else who needs saving from silence. But she hasn't done us a favour, because it is Classic FM, and they are playing fucking Vivaldi.

Up four flights of stairs, I'm introduced to Dr Dax, who extends a hand I cannot bear to touch. Her office looks like it's been ripped out of the pages of an interiors magazine. Mum and I sit in the velvet armchairs opposite her, and she spreads my notes across the glass coffee table, clicking her tongue. The room is tidy to the point of being a showroom. 'Lily,' Dr Dax says solemnly. 'We are here to discuss the fact that you are very sick. How do you feel?'

Nothing.

'You need to answer me. It's important I know how you are feeling, so we can decide on a treatment plan.'

'I'm sorry,' I say. 'I'm not trying to be difficult. I just . . . I just feel nothing.'

'I understand you used to be under the care of a Dr Finch. Your mother has said you don't wish to be seen by her anymore. We think it would be best if you were transferred to my care. Shall I keep her aware of your progress?'

'No,' I whisper. 'Please don't contact her.'

'As you wish,' says Dr Dax.

Looking at her mantelpiece, I realise the surfaces are not totally clear. Directly under a large Georgian mirror is a miniature bronze statue of a ballerina.

Dr Dax says the clinic doesn't offer inpatient stays. 'So I am going to admit you to Chesbury Hospital in London. I'll visit you there a few times a week.'

I'm supposed to be going to Chesbury tomorrow. I don't want to go. I don't like Dr Dax. I know Dr Finch is the only one who can help me; Dr Dax won't understand and might make things worse. I have to find Dr Finch. But how?

The problem can't be focused on right now, as I've spent

several hours today in Mum's company and am consumed by a flood of routines. I look at the time. It's almost 9.00pm, and I'm being admitted tomorrow at 10.00am.

Thirteen hours to change things.

I find the bottle of vodka that I've hidden under the heaps of mismatching pants and bras in my underwear drawer, unscrew the cap, and chug for a few seconds.

It lights a fire in my belly that courses through my blood and into my fingertips, which grip my pen and scribble down the routines more efficiently.

When I'm finished, I lie back on my bed and take a long glug. I lie still for a minute, feeling my thoughts eddying and crystallizing into a plan.

I will find Dr Finch and say sorry and ask her to help me. I don't know where she lives, but I know where she works. I will wait on the doorstep at Fieldness until she sees me.

I finish the vodka and hide the bottle in the drawer. Downstairs in the kitchen, Mum is cooking supper for her, Oliver, and me.

I can't go out the front door, because I'm not supposed to go anywhere by myself.

'I'm going outside for a cigarette,' I say.

'Okay, darling,' says Mum, stirring a pot of ratatouille and looking anxiously over her shoulder at me.

I head out into the back garden, shutting the back door. I don't have long. I disappear down the back passage and bolt over the gate, jumping down tipsily.

And I'm off: running like my life depends on it. There is a dull throbbing pain in my ankle where I hurt it on landing, but for now the vodka is working.

I need to get to the station, but if I take the main road Mum and Oliver might find me, so I'll have to navigate the back streets.

It's colder than I thought. My scraggy white cardigan isn't doing much.

I run in what I think is the direction of the station, until I realise I'm in an unrecognised cul-de-sac.

This is ridiculous. How can I be lost so close to home? I try to retrace my steps, but I can't work out where I came from. The road is spinning. The sky feels slanted.

I am.

Drunk.

I see two figures coming towards me. One, a man, is tall and lanky. The other is an outrageously fat woman.

'You look lost,' says the man, a black hoodie obscuring most of his face, though I see he has gold teeth, twinkling between syllables. 'Do you want to come home with us for a bit?'

Sirens wail in the distance. Are they coming for me?

I need to find Dr Finch. I need to . . . hide.

Is it better to go home with strangers but complete my mission, or fail here and now?

Just 15 minutes. Till the sirens are gone.

'O . . . K . . .'

The man says his name is Jay, his wife is Sharise.

They take me back to their block of flats. I realise it's the council estate that's a 15-minute drive from our house. I must have walked farther than I thought.

On the seventh floor, Jay pushes open a door with a nail where a number should be. I tumble into a smoke-filled sitting room, full of people crammed onto a sofa or lying on the floor.

'Come, come,' says Sharise. 'Excuse these fuckers! And you pissed as anything. You need some water.'

Jay grabs my arm and leads me through another door to a room with a double bed. Sharise comes in a second later, handing me a glass. The floor is a sea of empty fag packets, nail varnish pots, half-finished blister packs of pills, and dirty underwear.

Jay puts a CD on the player plugged in under the bed. I figured he'd go for heavy rap, but instead, the pained tinny notes of Avril Lavigne fill the room.

Hey, hey, you, you, I don't like your girlfriend!
No way, no way, I think you need a new one!

Sharise and Jay crash on the bed. I don't want to be in bed with them, so I squat on the floor. Jay lights up a joint, and I accept it for a few drags because I think it might make me less anxious. But the room swims even more, and I instantly regret it, because I know it will interfere with my mission. Sharise is making out with Jay. She pulls off her hair, which turns out to be a wig. The surprise of her bald scalp, littered with dark scabs, makes me gasp out loud.

I need to leave. But suddenly I am so sleepy I can't move. Did they put something in my water? Oh no, I'm accusing them of a crime even though it's probably the weed and my fault for saying yes. I am so judgmental, I am so quick to blame others for my own mistakes. What category should that go in? What category . . . should that . . .

I raise myself gently from the floor and peek over the edge of the bed. How long have I been out of it? Sharise and Jay are asleep, lying in bed, holding one another. I need to get out of here. The alarm clock on the floor reads 00.05.

I've missed the last train to Fenhurst. Idiot. My best bet will be waiting near the station until the train runs again.

I stand up quietly and creep out of the room. The sitting room has emptied. Where did everyone go? I've opened the front door when I feel a hand on my shoulder, and Jay's breath on my neck.

'Didn't enjoy your stay?'

My blood turns to ice. Sharise lumbers in behind him.

'Girl! You rude. We look after you, and you try to leave without saying good-bye. Why you do that? I don't like people who behave that way, do you, Jay?'

'No,' says Jay coldly, spinning me round and holding the neck of my T-shirt, pulling my face up to his. 'Are you scared? Do you think I'm going to hurt you? Do you think that's how I roll? Well, guess what. It's your lucky day. You're free to leave. You never hear of the kindness of strangers?'

'The lift's at the end,' shouts Sharise. I call it and turn around as the doors are closing. Sharise and Jay are still standing by their front door, staring at me.

The look in their eyes makes my skin crawl, and I will never forget it.

I walk along the middle of a deserted street.

I start to recognise things. I think I know where I'm going. Yes! Back on track!

But suddenly there's a police van behind me. I pick up the pace and start to run. Two policemen jump out and follow me on foot. Before they catch up, I know I can hide behind someone's dustbins, even though the dirt might kill me. But when I turn onto the new street, other police are ahead of me, and that's when I know it's a trap: I've been ambushed. They tell me my family has registered as me as a missing person at risk to herself.

They have been searching for me all night.

They put me in a police van.

I am thrashing around, no, don't take me, no, because excuse me but I have somewhere I need to be, actually—

And here comes the Blank Time, the part you'll rack your brains to remember when you're sober, but you never will, would you like to delete this footage? Voices telling you not to struggle, a half-developed image of your mother crying. Would you like to—

Yes.

Eyes open. Light, industrial in quality. Beeping. Body on a bed in a curtained cubicle. Body in a hospital gown, naked underneath.

Why? Where are my clothes? I try to sit up.

Mum to the left of me, hunched over in a plastic chair, making some horrendous attempt at sleep. She hears me stirring and turns to me.

Her face is puffy—like someone's been at it with an air pump. Under each eye, a slick of purple.

'Thank god you're okay,' she whispers, cheeks streaked with tears. 'Thank god you're okay. What were you *thinking*?'

Sometimes, there just are no replies.

But sometimes, people need replies.

'DON'T YOU LOVE US?' she cries. 'Don't you give a shit about us?

Who is us?

'Dad, Oliver, and I have been out all night looking for you. Dad was searching the park. He thought you had gone there. He really thought you were dead.'

Oh.

'We've been besides ourselves. So now I'm asking you, what's your problem? Don't you love us?'

'I do, I do.'

'So why are you behaving like this? They had to sedate you last night! Why are you—'

Oliver comes through the curtain. He tells Mum to calm down; he says it's not helping.

'We've been really worried, Lily,' he says. 'We're so relieved we've found you.'

'I'm sorry,' I say. 'Can we go?'

'The doctor will need to discharge you, I think.' Mum sighs. 'Once he does, we'll go home, pack a bag, and then I'll take you to Chesbury.'

We wait in agonizing quiet—the loud silence of 1,000 shiny arrows ready to be fired.

22

Urine Test

When we arrive at Chesbury Hospital, and after leaving my stuff in my room, Mum says we should have a look around, so we traipse off to explore.

In the lounge, there's a surprise. My mum stops in her tracks, and a middle-aged woman lying on the couch jumps up like a jack-in-the-box.

'Helena!' She smiles manically and waves her hands in a frantic fanning motion.

'Paula . . . Hi!' replies Mum, before turning to a younger girl on the sofa next to Paula.

'Are you here with your daughter too?'

'Nope! Haha! I'm one of the nutters. Surprise!'

'Lily . . .' Mum turns to me, possibly uncertain whether confidentiality applies to this sort of meet-and-greet, before seeming to have a fuck-it-who-cares moment.

'This is Paula. We used to work together in the practice. Paula is an architect.'

'Oh, hi, Paula! Lovely to meet you,' I stumble.

'How's things?' asks Mum.

'Oh great, really great.' Paula grins, but her eyes look hollow.

The conversation flags, as everyone takes a minute to acknowledge that 'great' probably wasn't the right word. Then, thankfully, Paula says, 'Well, actually, the truth is, I have bipolar disorder. And I've been really ill. I've basically been in and out of hospital for the last 10 years. I'm having a bad patch again. I maxed out my credit card and bought a ton of Macs and iPads with money I didn't have. So I'm back here recovering. You must have known I was ill—I was always the loopy one at the office party! You should go. It's not so bad here. I'll look after Lily, don't worry!'

Mum is hesitant, but takes Paula's instructions nonetheless. She hugs me and goes to the nursing station to tell them she's off. I run back to my room because my window overlooks the car park. I watch her driving away in her silver Beetle. She said she loved me earlier, no matter what. But how can she, when I've ruined so much?

I wonder whether she will come back.

I acknowledge I am a Patient at the Hospital and agree to its rules and regulations.

'Melanie, one of the nurses, will give you a tour later,' says the head nurse, Barbara, a robust, no-nonsense type. 'She'll show you the art room, the studio, and the gym.'

I picture the timetable:

8.30am: continental breakfast
10.00am: Tai chi
11.00am: group therapy
12.00pm: luncheon (please notify the head chef of any dietary requirements)
1.00pm: music therapy
2.00pm: walking therapy or aqua-therapy
3.00pm: artistic expression

4.00pm: yoga and meditation
5.00pm: dance and physical expression workshop
6.00pm: lecture, 'Building Bridges'
7.00pm: dinner (please see menu)
10.00pm: the only person in the whole building who hasn't gone bonkers kills herself. The other patients cheer . . .

A nurse says they will need blood and urine samples. 'Why?' I ask.

'We need to make sure there are no illegal substances in your body. It's normal protocol when a patient arrives.'

'But that's not why I'm here.' Perhaps she has made a mistake. 'I don't have a drug problem,' I clarify.

'I don't make the rules, sugar,' the nurse says. 'Now get back to your room.'

I do not want to have my blood taken. Imagine all the drug users here who've caught diseases; what if they mix up our needles? I am certain I'm about to contract HIV and die.

'Bloodz!'

A skinny Polish woman enters my room, the observation room near the nurses' station, swinging a yellow hazardous-waste bucket.

'Sleeve up!' she commands.

I roll my sleeve up and look away. No one can say I am not trying to comply. I feel her jab me and imagine the HIV virus entering my body, swimming through my veins like tiny piranhas. Oh well, I sigh. You tried to kill yourself: surely you can't care that much about getting ill?

Melanie comes in.

'Is it time for the guided tour?' I ask hopefully.

'Not yet, hon. Come do a pee in the pot for me first.'

When I ask if it can be done later, she shakes her head. 'Not much point you doing it once you've detoxed, is there?'

'I'm not on drugs.'

'Mmm.'

I try a new approach.

'I just don't want to give my pee away to anyone, because it belongs to me.'

'That's a new one.'

'So I don't have to do it?'

'Just get in the bathroom, girl!'

I make my way towards the toilet opposite my room, shutting the door as per normal when—BAM—quick as a flash, Melanie jabs her foot in front of the door so I can't shut it.

'Is there a problem?' I whisper, a cold sweat prickling across my back.

'Yeah. I'm coming in too. Otherwise you could just use someone else's urine, couldn't you?'

'Someone else's pee? How would I even—'

'Tubes, water bottles, your mouth—people are creative.'

Shutting the door behind her, she folds her arms and stares me down as I lower my pants and place myself on the seat. The odds of me peeing in front of someone are slim to none.

'How long does it take, girl?'

'I can't do it with someone in here. I don't need to go anyway.'

'Okay, fair enough, drink some water and you can try again in half an hour.'

I drink six cups, though I know it's futile. I think I'm constitutionally unable to pee in front of anyone. Melanie escorts me again.

And again.

And again.

By now five hours have passed, and I understand why she's

suspicious.

'Look, if you've taken drugs, that's okay. It wouldn't be the first time round here, that's for sure. You just need to be honest with us, okay? What was it you took? Go for a pee, we'll run some tests so we can find out how to help you.'

I shake my head and look at the floor.

'Okay, play the hard game. You wanna be like that, fine. You're only hurting yourself. I've got all day.'

They peek through a small inspection window in my door every 10 minutes to see what I'm up to.

I'm told to go along to a 'community meeting' in 'the lounge.' Since I've only been here a few hours, I don't have anything to contribute, but they encourage me to listen.

'For those of you who don't know,' begins Barbara, looking at me, 'community meeting is where we meet to discuss any . . . issues . . . and other things that are on our mind. So, who would like to start?'

A pause. For a second I think this might be one of those awkward meetings where everyone just pretends they aren't there. But then the circus breaks out, and I realise how wrong I was. The pause was just the stockpiling of breath required for a verbal marathon:

'I want a remote for the TV—'

'I want fucking caffeinated coffee!'

'—it's so dull having to get up every time you want to change the channel.'

'And caffeinated tea too! Don't forget all the people who drink tea!'

'There should be a TV rota because—'

'We urgently need more board games.'

'—it's really unfair how Celie hogs it all the time—'

'A remote would cost what—a tenner? And how much are we paying to stay here?'

'—cos no one else wants to watch back-to-back *Sixteen and Pregnant*.'

'We should be able to order in food!'

'Like I want to play Mouse Trap? Who remembers Mouse Trap? I'm so fucking bored of Monopoly.'

'And Risk!'

'The nurses need to stop waking me up in the night for checks—of course I'm still bloody there—'

'And Operation!'

'And sandwiches! In the day! Just on the ward—'

'—I'm not fucking Houdini.'

'Longer fag breaks!'

'—because you know, people get hungry between meals.'

'All right! All right, everyone, well, I think we've got lots of suggestions there and I'll pass them on. Now'—she puts on what sounds like a nursery-teacher voice, and for a second I think she might be about to read us a story: 'Annabel sat very patiently with her hand up while all of you were making your thoughts known, so I'm going to give her a chance to talk, and we're all going to listen.'

She taps her ears encouragingly, in case some of us have forgotten where our auditory organs are located. Annabel begins.

'Well, it's just like I woke up the other morning and I actually have really low blood sugar levels so I knew I needed something to eat right then and there and that I wouldn't have the energy to get out of bed and get anything, so I rang my alarm bell. Anyway, no one came, and meanwhile my blood sugar was diminishing. So luckily I had some squirty honey in my room, but if I hadn't had that, I think something very serious could have happened. So I'm just raising this as a suggestion that I think it would be a good idea if all the alarm bells were checked to see it they're working so that I'm not put in danger again. And, yeah. That's all I had to say.'

Barbara nods wearily. 'Okay, Annabel, we'll see if we can get the alarms checked. Right, then! That's community meeting dismissed.'

Back in my room, my bladder feels like it's going to explode.

Melanie sighs. 'Surely you need to go now.' 'I do, I really do, but I . . .'

This is our sixth attempt. Every fiber in me wants to go, yet I can't. I try 'pushing,' but I'm not sure that's even right for peeing. I feel like crying.

Maybe they could use my tears instead? I don't even really want to give them those.

'Drink five more cups of water,' instructs Melanie. It turns out she doesn't have all day, because her shift ends at 6.00pm. She is replaced by a new nurse whose job is to make sure I don't urinate unattended.

Unlike Melanie, Justine doesn't escort me to the toilet every 30 minutes. She is Jamaican, and more laissez-faire in her approach to urine collection.

'You wanna go pee pee? No? Okay. When it happen, it happen.' She shrugs.

I feel calmer under the new pee regime. I stay in my room and try to read a book, feigning oblivion to Justine's six glances an hour through the observation slat. I hope that pretending not to notice someone doesn't make me a liar.

Right now I am preoccupied by four categories:

BITCH
LIAR
BODILY FUNCTIONS
and
PERVERT.
I recite the letters:
NS, D, BHB, E.

Here are the actions I must account for:

BITCH:
1. <u>N</u>OT GOING TO TOILET: Melanie is going to think I'm a brat who wants to cause trouble by not going to the toilet when told, in a pathetic act of rebellion.

2. <u>S</u>MILE: On the way to the toilet a patient passed me in the corridor and gave me a smile, but I was busy thinking about going to the toilet, and by the time I had realised she was smiling at me and made the right face to smile back, she had already walked past. It looked like I had snubbed her, which may make her feel sad.

LIAR:
1. <u>D</u>RUGS: Melanie will think I'm lying about not taking drugs—otherwise why would I not go to the toilet?

BODILY FUNCTIONS:
1. <u>B</u>REATHING: Was I breathing too deeply when Melanie was in the toilet with me? Did she hear because it was so quiet and think it was gross?

2. <u>H</u>AIRY LEGS: Melanie was watching me when I pulled my pants down. There was a bit of hair on the top of my legs because I haven't shaved since I was in Ireland. She probably thought I was unkempt.

3. <u>B</u>ODY ODOUR: When I stood up to wash my hands in the sink, Melanie didn't move from by the door, meaning we were inches apart. What if I have a really horrible smell to my body that I can't smell but she could?

PERVERT:

1. <u>E</u>YE CONTACT WITH MELANIE: My eyes made contact with Melanie as I was sitting on the toilet. What if she thinks I was aroused by being in the toilet with my pants down in front of another girl and was making eye contact to see if she was up for it?

Eventually Justine knocks. 'It's 11 o'clock, girlie. My notes say ya haven't peed for 12 hours. That can't be healthy, girl! Where you putting ya pee?'

She pretends to look under my bed, which unnerves me.

'Okay, here's the thing,' I say, wondering how best to explain the situation. 'I don't want to give someone my pee, and I definitely can't pee in front of anyone, because that's just too gross. But I need to go so badly, it's possible I could compromise. If you wait outside and let me go by myself, I will . . .' I take a deep breath and summon my courage. 'I will let you have my pee.'

'Ohhhh! The girl just wants some privaceee! Well, why didn't ya say in the first place?' Justine laughs with a hearty belly gurgle.

Unlike Melanie, Justine clearly isn't aware of the ingenuity of patients. I run to the toilet and give them what they want. When I present Justine with the pot, she pats me on the back. 'Now that weren't so hard, were it, girl?' she chortles, skipping off with her hard-won prize.

The day ends with a message from on high: Dr Dax is changing my medication.

I ask Barbara if she knows the reason for the change. 'Do I look like a doctor, hon?' comes the reply. 'It's probably just a trial thing. You can ask your doctor when she comes.'

I go to breakfast with Annabel, but don't eat anything. She regales me with stories of her holiday home in Malta, and I try to nod in the right places. Afterwards, it's back to my room. I'm soon joined by Tilly, a wide-eyed 'therapy coordinator' who has come to help me organise my time. She hands me a list of activities.

'These are all the things you could do. Circle the things that interest you, and I'll put together a personalised timetable for you. You'll be assigned a private therapist, who will see you twice a week for CBT.'

'Do I have to do any of them?'

'Yes,' she chirps. 'Otherwise you're not complying with your treatment. Go on. I won't watch.'

'Okay . . .' I look down at the list. I like walking, so I circle 'Group walk in Bawton Park.'

'Oh, you can't do that one! Walks are reserved for our safer patients.'

I settle for art therapy and hand back the sheet.

'You have to choose more than one. What about the drama workshops or yoga? You have OCD, don't you? Okaaay . . . we also have a CBT group for OCD patients once a week.'

I have to choose a few more. By now I've built up so many routines, primarily about her proximity to me (she's sitting on my bed), that I just want to get rid of her. I circle some activities at random.

'The stress discussion group, family support session, depression discussion group, and free time in the art room! Great choices!'

With a flourish, she whips the paper away and strides off in the direction of the door, turning around to give me a wink. 'In the next couple of days we'll organise some sessions with a private therapist, and Dr Dax will visit a few times a week. I'll have your timetable made up by tomorrow! You're going to love it!'

Tilly closes the door, and I lie back on my bed, trying to neutralise the fear that I had bad breath when I spoke to her by reassuring myself that since I've already brushed my teeth seven times today, that's unlikely.

I skip lunch, and stay where I am all day. At around 7.00pm, I venture into the kitchen to make myself a cup of decaffeinated tea.

A girl with black hair turns around, and I realise she smiled at me earlier when I didn't react quickly enough to smile back. I make up for it now by giving a really good smile, and I feel like an *IDIOT*.

'Hey,' she says. 'I'm Frankie. Are you a smoker? You look like a smoker. Want to go and have one with me when you've made your drink?'

I haven't had a fag in over a day. I've been too scared to leave my room or ask where the smoking area is.

'Okay,' I say. She steps back and indicates with an elaborate flourish of her arm that it's my turn to use the hot water tank. She stands impressively still, but it's the sort of stillness that makes no promises as to how long it will stay that way. She squints her eyes and looks me up and down without saying anything.

She reminds me of a cat.

We walk into a snow-covered courtyard in the centre of the building. We sit on the bench and watch twirls of smoke float into the night sky.

Frankie is 32, but acts 10 years younger. She tells me she's been shuttled in and out of mental hospitals since boarding school, and suffers from bipolar disorder. She is also a part-time heroin user. Frankie is in a senior position at an oil giant, but you wouldn't know it. She giggles like a schoolgirl when her boss comes to visit, playing the too-ill-for-company-right-now card.

Early in my stay, her 50-year-old boyfriend Archie, whom she met in a previous rehab, comes to see her. He is also a heroin user, and the staff disapprove of him visiting. We all sit in the garden chain-smoking our way through a pack of cigarettes. Frankie turns to Archie and looks at him lovingly, blowing smoke on his face with a little smile.

I leave them to have some quality time and toddle off back to my room. I assume the reading position, sitting upright and holding a book in front of my face so that the nurses won't bother me, because reading is considered a healthy use of time that needn't be interrupted, whereas staring into space is not. I'm coming to the end of an hour-long loop of routines about what happened while smoking outside when a flushed Melanie bursts through my door without knocking, meaning I'll have to start again.

'Have you seen Frankie? You were hanging out with her earlier, right?'

'I was with her earlier, but I haven't seen her since I came back to my room.'

'Okay,' she garbles and runs off in the other direction.

Meds are at 9.00pm, and I notice that my pills have been changed again. Since Dr Dax has yet to explain yesterday's change, I think there might have been a mistake. The man dispensing, who I haven't seen before, tells me it's best for me to take them, and that there definitely hasn't been a mistake.

A grey-faced Frankie is pulled in the door by nurses a little after that. It turns out she'd sneaked out and gone home with Archie to do some heroin.

I'm getting water from the dispenser in the main corridor when she arrives.

I am relieved to discover that I can still feel sadness.

23

Loser, Friend

'They wanted to move me to the addicts' ward,' Frankie explains to me with her mouth full over breakfast the next day. 'But I wouldn't let them. You're the only one I like here, so we have to stay on the same ward.'

I smile, wide it probably makes me look like a friendless creep.

'Have you been to any of the stuff on your timetable?' Frankie asks. I shake my head because I don't want to talk with my mouth full, adding **S**TUPID MUTE to my list, also in *LOSER*.

'Neither, it's a load of bollocks!' she declares. 'Tell you what— today we're going to have fun!'

'What sort of fun?' I reply, trying not to sound too reserved, because that would be three things in *LOSER* in less than a minute.

'I dunno! We'll find things to do. There's loads of stuff to do in an old place like this—it's like a castle! We should explore.'

'But you're on five-minute checks . . .'

'Don't worry,' she grins. 'I'm a pro.'

Frankie informs today's nurse, Kelsie, that we are going for a cigarette, and Kelsie in turn informs us that she will be watching us from the window.

Out in the garden, I'm in for another surprise. A willowy, pale-faced girl with dyed blonde hair and a narrow angular face is puffing away on a cigarette. With a jolt, I realise we were at school together. She was in the year above: sassy and popular. Now here she is with bandaged wrists, looking like death.

'Hey.' I struggle. 'It's Chloe, isn't it?'

'Yeah.'

Too late, I realise people here don't want to be recognised, and I hate myself for handling the situation tactlessly. Frankie, on the other hand, is oblivious.

'Oh, cooool, babes. What boarding school were you guys at?'

'Hambledon,' we answer, in sync.

'Haha! No way! I have a stepsister there. Do you know Katie Moore?'

'I didn't know her. But I remember her name,' I say.

'She's okay . . . ,' continues Frankie. 'But her mum, my supposed stepmum, is a BIATCH! She totally ruined our family. And I'm not even joking. Chloe, you, me, and Lily probably have so many friends in common. Haha! Funny, isn't it? Us three, all graduates from the best private schools in the country, headed straight to Chesbury University. Boarding really does fuuuuuck you up!'

Chloe gives a thin smile.

'Okay . . . we're off now!' says Frankie. 'See ya later!'

Shutting the door to the garden behind us, I give Chloe a little wave. Frankie has no time for good-byes; she is marching along the corridor.

'We've been gone for about seven minutes, so they'll be looking for me already. Our nursing station is up those stairs . . . so we need to go this way to avoid being spotted.'

We sprint down corridors, past patients getting creative in the art room, and via various 'engaged' rooms in which people are being made better by talking, before hurtling through a door, down some stairs, and through another door. That door must be a magic portal, because suddenly the buzz of the hospital is far behind.

'Woah,' says Frankie, looking down at a tiny staircase that leads to a lower level. I dash down it, giggling, keen to prove that I am not a *LOSER*.

'Come on, Frankie! Look at this old wooden door!'

Frankie arrives at my side, panting.

'It's gonna be locked. I know it.' I laugh.

Loser.
Loser.
Loser!

'Push it!' Frankie is right behind me now, shoving into me as I grip the door handle.

We tumble headfirst onto the carpet.

We appear to be in an old doctor's office that looks like it hasn't been used for ages. Over the years, stuff must have just stacked up as staff used the room for storage. To the average person it might look like a dump, but to two bored inpatients, it's a treasure trove.

Frankie is spinning round on a swivel chair behind the desk with a notepad and pen she has found somewhere.

'Now, Lily,' she drawls in a thick German accent, pretending to make notes, 'I'm going to give you your diagnosis! You're batshit crazzzzyyyyyyy!'

I'm rooting through a box that turns out to be full of hundreds of yellow journals from the British College of Psychiatrists, dated 1950–1990.

'Frankie, shut up, someone's going to hear us! Quick, come and look what I've found!'

Frankie crawls round a gilded mirror that for some unknown reason has been plonked in the middle of the room, and crouches next to me.

'Look at all these old journals!'

'OMG!' squeals Frankie. 'Well done you! Bedtime reading for a month!'

But Frankie can't wait till bedtime. She pulls out journals at random and flicks through them so quickly it reminds me of fast-forwarding through videotapes when I was little. The journals are filled with garishly coloured adverts about how fantastic pills are. A cartoon helicopter promises that Parnate is a Depression Lifter. A few pages later, a paper ticket superimposed on a crowd at a train station says that Orap offers a first-class return from hospital to society. Then there are people in fun-fair mirrors who are wiggly, short, and tall, and the caption says that 'depressed people come in all shapes and sizes. . . . Nearly all of them will respond well to PROTHIADEN.'

'These adverts for pills are classic!' Frankie laughs. 'The pharmaceutical industry would never be allowed to advertise like this these days. Do you think these things are worth anything? Like, are they collectable?'

'Maybe. . . . I want to read the studies in them while I'm here; they look really interesting. Let's take some,' I say, with more confidence than I feel. 'It's not like anyone wants them.'

'Agreed. And shit! Look at the time. That new nurse is going to be going mad!'

We hide the journals underneath my parka, which I put on to go for a cigarette. It looks like I'm about to give birth to a square baby.

'Why do you only want the ones from 1981?' Frankie asks.

'Well, I want 12 months' worth. A set.'

'Is that an OCD thing?'

'I don't think so. It's just logical.'

'K babes, I get ya,' says Frankie, grabbing journals at random and flinging them into the handbag she takes everywhere with her. 'You're right. We need to go now.'

I open the door a crack and peek round to make sure no one is coming.

'Coast clear!'

Out we dart, looping round the upper levels of the hospital to avoid going via the main nursing stations from other wards and being spotted—somehow, Frankie knows where they all are— before descending again to our ward.

'Where've you been?' demands Kelsie, drumming her fingers against the wall.

'We were in the art room, making pictures' says Frankie without a second's hesitation.

'Where are the pictures, then?'

'They're on the art rack, drying, because we painted them. Duh!'

I nod enthusiastically, hoping I'm a good partner in crime.

'Oh!' says Kelsie, smiling. 'Well, that's lovely. Really, lovely. . . . See you later, then.'

Suitably appeased, Kelsie shoots off in the other direction. I tell Frankie I'm going to dump the journals in my cupboard and start reading some of them. Frankie says 'No stress, man,' which I think means 'Okay,' and heads back towards the lounge.

I tiptoe past the nursing station, desperate not to engage in conversation with another human. I hide all the journals in my room, except for November 1981, which I clamber into bed with. I'm gambling on the fact that the nurses won't know what it is, and will just assume I'm reading another book.

I lean back on the pillows and assume the reading position,

staring with intent at a page advert that is filled by a child's painting of a crying face on a stick body titled 'My mum.' The face has eyes with paint drips running down from them like tears, and a big pink frown. In the corner the artist has signed 'Cordelia W. age 4.' Then underneath that, a line of text reads: 'Which antidepressant is highly effective and avoids the tricyclic hangover? See next page for prescribing information.'

It has been an hour and 50 minutes since I've been by myself. I've enjoyed hanging out with Frankie, but the routines have piled up as usual, and now I'm at bursting point. When I spend uninterrupted time with other people, a dam builds in my head. It can hold the words back for a while, but at some point they'll surge free and overflow, and there will be chaos.

Lying back, I try to sort out the words.

On the morning of day five, someone knocks on my door. I look up and see Tilly through the observation slat.

'Lily,' she announces, marching into the room, 'we need to talk. The nurses tell me you haven't been going to your activities. Remember what I said about not complying with treatment?' Big smile. 'Well, if you don't go, I will have to tell Dr Dax, and we might have to move you to a more secure ward.'

'That's true,' I say, 'but you also haven't stuck to the timetable. I haven't been assigned a therapist for CBT yet.'

Tilly's smile falters. Frankie's face pops up at the observation slat. She's pulling faces and wagging her finger like Tilly. I try not to laugh.

'We are trying to arrange the best possible treatment for you at a difficult time. At the moment, that means going to your activities.'

'But none of those activities work for me. They all involve sitting in a large group of people for long periods of time, and that sort of situation sends my OCD into a whir.'

'What about yoga?'

'Yoga is hell. I just lie there doing stuff in my head and getting stressed because they're telling me to pretend I'm on some mountain that doesn't exist. Maybe it would be great if I was better, but right now it's the last thing I want to be doing.'

'The nurses will keep me informed. Think about it.' She pats my shoulder, which sends a ripple of aftershocks through my body.

Will traces of my SHOULDER be left on her palm?

Tilly turns to leave the room. Frankie's face disappears, only to fly through my door 30 seconds later.

'Morning! Breakfast time! So you have to go to your activities?'

'You eavesdropper!'

'Noooo, it's not like that, I'm just looking out for you!' She grabs the personalised timetable from my hands. 'Oooh! You have art today! So do I. We'll go together.'

Jenny's voice wafts through the room like a relaxation DVD.

'Use whatever medium you like. There's Plasticine, crayons, pencils, or paint. The choice is yours.'

There are six of us around the table. A fat woman from another ward stares vacantly into space, rolling the pink Plasticine around slowly.

To my left, an ex-military guy called Sam, who is being treated for post-traumatic stress disorder, is using the yellow Plasticine to make handguns.

On my right, Frankie clutches crayons in the air, raring to go. A pink-haired girl called Delia is getting her brushes and paint palette ready.

Finally, there's Amy. Amy was from Kansas, but now lives in Fulham with her husband and two kids. Her problems mainly centre round the fear that her face doesn't look as good as those of her mum peers. She also finds being class rep stressful, and is increasingly alienated by mum-to-mum playground politics.

'Basically,' she summarises, 'I am so goddamn sick of tiger mothers getting me down. Ya know?'

Jenny nods sympathetically, then says, 'Today's theme is confidence. I would like you all to draw, make, or create something that expresses how you feel about confidence. You have 30 minutes.'

Frankie leans close and whispers to me: 'Challenge—I bet I can make something more clichéd than you.'

'Oh, you are so on,' I hiss back.

Frankie draws herself as half Lucifer and half Gabriel. I draw a gawky human puppet being pulled up from a curled ball to standing: the taller she gets, the uglier she becomes.

'Oh, wow, that is breathtaking, Lily,' says Jenny, when the time limit is up. 'Can you describe your work to the group?'

'Uh, yes, I, uh . . . I think . . . Too much confidence is ugly. Yes, that's what I think. That's why I made this.'

Frankie has pulled her sweater halfway over her face and is trying to disguise her laughter as a cough. She's not doing a very good job.

'Gosh!' interjects Amy. 'That is just one of the most powerful things I've ever heard. Too much confidence is ugly.'

She shakes her head in disbelief. 'I'm going to write that down. Ya know, I might get it printed on a canvas and hang it in my hallway. Too much confidence is ugly . . .'

24

Skating

This morning, when I wake up, I picture some white skating boots and my head. For hours, all I can see is the tip of the blade smacking into the back of my skull, gradually chipping away at the bone until blood spurts everywhere. I convince myself I will never be able to think of anything else for the rest of my life, and the thought swells and magnifies.

Outside, I can hear Dr Dax stalking the corridors. She swoops in on a cloud of sickly perfume and designer clothing, perches on my bed, and tries to chat about whether I am enjoying my stay.

I cannot cope.

I scream at her and ask her why she keeps changing my medication without explanation. My *SPOILED* category is going into overdrive, but for once, I don't care.

'I can't stop eating!' I gesture round my room towards the sweet and chocolate wrappers littering the floor and the stack of crisp packets in the bin. I wave the banana I'm halfway through eating at her like a crazed ape girl. 'I never used to be like this! Those pills make me eat everything in sight, and Frankie said it's true because she's been on them and you stop knowing when you're full. And why have I had no proper CBT? Dr Finch said that's the only behavioural therapy for OCD that works. Why did I spend yesterday afternoon listening to dumb people defining the

word *stress* on a big whiteboard with a spider diagram, and why
did I have to make a 'worry tree' in depression class?'

Dr Dax replies evenly, 'I'm sorry you feel some negativity
towards the service you have received.'

'It's YOUR fault!' I howl. 'YOUR fault I can't stop thinking
about ice skates, because this treatment is WRONG. I wouldn't
be thinking about ice skates if it weren't for YOU changing my
medication and making me sit in huge groups of people and
I FEEL ALL WRONG IN MY HEAD AND IT'S WORSE
THAN BEFORE. And now you're sitting here making me feel
angry, and all I can think about is ICE SKATES HITTING
MY HEAD—'

I picture another white boot taking aim. I wince. The
thought becomes so vivid, I hear my skull crack.

'Lily,' Dr Dax says slowly, 'have you ever considered the fact
that you might be psychotic?'

'I'm not! Dr Finch said another doctor would say that! It's an
intrusive thought, which of course you don't know anything
about, because I'm not sure you even know what OCD is. GO
AWAY!'

'As you wish.'

Dr Dax leaves.

A nurse comes in with a thimble-size paper cup of water and
a pill.

'Take this.'

'I don't want to.'

'It's best you take it.'

I am too tired to fight. I sit up to swallow the pill and lie back
down. Everything becomes wobbly and slower, and I feel a dull
numbness setting in.

I sink down in the bed and sleep.

Frankie bursts in around 4.00pm.

'Oh my gawd can you pull yourself together I've had such a boring day without you!'

I sit up groggily

'Okay, it's fun time now. So I did some exploring while you were drugged up. Turns out there's this whole layer of offices in the attic that we didn't know about.'

We wait for the nurses' changeover time. Engrossed in paperwork, they don't see us walk off the ward. We walk with purpose up to the attic. The offices aren't locked. Once inside, Frankie starts rifling through drawers.

'Holy shit, look, office scissors! Tell you what, they could slash some wrists in the wrong hands! It's pretty terrible that they've just been left out like this, I mean, imagine if someone who self-harms found them.' She furrows her forehead in concern. 'They could be useful though, if we're careful. I'm going to take them.'

'But you don't self-harm, and neither do I, so what use do we have for scissors?'

'For collaging.'

Frankie and I have started making collages out of magazines on our ward. And she's right. It would be a lot quicker if we didn't tear all the pages by hand.

I'm sweeping the desks, when I notice a yellow Post-it on the wall and realise what the numbers written on it mean.

'Frankie!' I'm so excited I grab her arm, before regretting it, because unsolicited contact could make me a *PERVERT.* 'Frankie, stop!'

I take the Post-it from the wall and wave it at her.

'Look! You know how we never knew how to get through

all those doors with codes? Well, this is the door code. They've written it on a Post-it note so they don't forget it! Let's find out what we're missing!'

We dash down to a separate wing, trying to look inconspicuous when passing orderlies. Frankie punches in the code. The door swings open onto a corridor, but neither of us have the guts to go down it, for fear of meeting any mad people. Change direction then—back where we came from and then up a few flights of stairs and along a corridor, a new door beckons. This one isn't coded, and it opens onto a staircase, which we run up. At the top, there is a white door to a fire escape. More to the point, a white door, ajar.

We cannot believe it. Here, right in front of us, is a chink of real life.

'Bingo!' I squeal. 'Where should we go?!'

I'm still not allowed to join the walks in the park, or go on an escorted walk to the corner shop, because I am 'too high-risk.' Frankie has no chance of being allowed outside after her previous escapade. The only fresh air we've had has been in the outdoor smoking area.

'Lily, you know how pissed off you were about your Coke?'

Three days ago, it was decided I was drinking too much Diet Coke, and the six-packs Mum had brought for me were confiscated. They are now being held under lock and key in the nursing station, and I get dispensed one a day by knocking on their door and groveling.

'There's a corner shop down the road,' Frankie says in a rush. 'I know because the nurses escorted me there with the others to buy fags when I was still allowed out. We'll go and get you a ton of Coke, and then you can drink it secretly.'

We push the door open. It's only 6.00pm, but it's already

dark. I inhale the swirling wind in private ecstasy. We creep down the fire escape onto a thin layer of snow.

We plod to the corner shop, shivering in our T-shirts. I thought the man behind the till would spot us crazies a mile off, but he doesn't give us a second look. For the first time since my arrival, I feel like a normal human. Frankie, whose trusted handbag is at hand, pays for as much Coke as we can carry.

We could escape for good now, get a cab to the airport and buy one-way tickets to America (Frankie says she has enough money on her card to pay for tickets); we could go clubbing, or just kill ourselves like we wanted to in the first place.

But we don't. We turn around, walk back to the fire escape, and go quietly through the door and back to our rooms like nothing has happened.

'Fuck it!' yells Paula. 'The remote doesn't work again! I don't know why they can't just get some bloody batteries. It's not like we're not paying enough to stay here!'

'How much does it cost to stay here?' I ask, trying to sound offhand. I know it isn't cheap, but I've never managed to ascertain the figure.

'Like £900 a day, I think. That's right, isn't it, Annabel?'

'Something like that, yeah,' she replies distantly, munching on some loose skin around her forefinger.

My stomach drops. Since my arrival, my medication has been messed with so much I feel like a human experiment, and I haven't had a single one-to-one CBT session. I've basically mucked around with Frankie all day, smoked, and watched TV, all at a cost of just under £900 a day. I need to get out of here. It's time for a distress flare.

I go back to my room, take my mobile out of the drawer,

and write Dr Finch an e-mail asking if I can talk to her. I hit send—*Mayday, Mayday, Mayday*: a blast of red sparks sent up into the sky.

It is 1.18pm, and I am expecting a call from Dr Finch at 1.30. Based on past experience, she will ring at 1.35 or 1.45. In preparation for this momentous occasion, I have finished all of the day's routines so I can give the conversation my full attention. Unfortunately, I time everything wrong. I finish my routines at 1.06, which leaves around half an hour for new routines to generate. In a desperate attempt to stop this, I revert to Upper Ock tactics. I go to the hospital gym and set the running machine to full pelt.

For the first time ever, Dr Finch rings ahead of schedule.

My phone, which I've slotted in the treadmill's cup holder, is buzzing. Fuck.

I panic, pressing the emergency stop while reaching to take the call. The machine drops from 12 miles per hour to a standstill, and I fly off the back. My mobile spins across the waxed floor. I crawl over and grab it, cradling it in my hands like an injured baby bird. I dash into the corridor, collapse into a sweaty heap, press green, and put the receiver to my ear.

'Hi, it's Lily,' I pant.

'Hi, Lily. It's me, Dr Finch. You said you wanted to talk?'

'I've got to get out of here. I've just found out how much it costs, and I feel awful because that is a crazy amount of money to spend on this treatment. And I was wrong. You're the only one who can help me. And I can't just walk out, so you have to get me transferred. I'm sorry about all the stuff I said. I didn't mean it. I was just . . . Everything was messed up. If you take me back, I promise to be good and do everything you say and—'

'Wait, wait, slow down. You can't see me at Fieldness—the inpatient unit has closed down now. But I also practice at the Leneston Hospital in Ashleaves. You could be admitted there. Are you sure this is what you want, though?'

'Yes, yes, definitely.'

'Okay. I'll get it sorted. I'll talk to your parents and the hospital and arrange a transfer.'

'Okay, thank you. Thank you so much. Bye.'

'Bye, Lily.'

The line goes dead. Relief and joy pulse through my body, surging to my heart like an electric current earthing itself.

Now all I have to do is tell Frankie.

I am waiting on the porch with my bag when my mum pulls up in the Beetle. The nurses don't come to see me off, but Frankie and Delia do. Hugging is obligatory. 'Good-bye!' I call from the front seat, to which Delia grins and replies 'Ciao.'

'I don't do good-byes. This isn't good-bye,' says Frankie, the smile fading from her face. She turns around, grabs Delia by the arm, and walks back into the grand entrance hall. The double glass doors swing shut behind her, and I watch until she disappears.

I will miss Frankie. She was constant and unavoidable in a way even my routines couldn't destroy. She fizzed with life and a lust for fun. She stretched her hand out to a version of myself I thought I'd lost forever, held me tight, and then, when I least expected it, pulled me back from the brink.

25

Ashleaves

In the Beetle with my mum, I feel my stomach pancake-flip. I want to yell to stop the car, pull over, turn around, go home, or head in any direction that isn't bound for Dr Finch.

We travel in companionable silence, leaving London behind with a jolt as we hit the M25. Around us, a cloudless cool blue morning potters on with its business, oblivious to the nervous chill evoked in me by the route I associate with returning to school and visits to Dr Finch.

It's strange—wanting but not wanting. Wanting: to run to Dr Finch and spend forever with her. Let me orbit you, I could say; be my star and let me go round and round until either I'm better or you love me too. Not wanting: to see her and glimpse the truth. She doesn't care for me in that way. She can't, she never will. She sees me for what I am, every flaw apparent. Lifts me close to her face, but only for scientific inspection. I'm her bug in a glass paperweight, held fast whether it likes it or not.

And yet still hoping, that maybe, one day . . .

Ashleaves offers a brief attempt at something resembling a city, but it's over as soon as it has begun. Soon we find ourselves on a steep road that cuts through fields, winding up to a gate that opens onto a ridiculously long driveway, which points like an arrow towards Dr Finch's second home, the Leneston Hospital. It looks like it was probably a cheery country house until quite recently.

A blonde woman on reception directs us up a floor. We arrive on the ward, where head nurse Bob introduces himself and shows us my new room; I let Mum do the talking and nod. We have to walk past the nursing station, the door of which is open.

I glimpse Dr Finch perched against one of the desks in a red wool V-neck and brown pencil skirt, sporting characteristically untamed hair. She is chatting intently to one of the other nurses, but her gaze shifts subtly to us as we walk past. I cannot meet her eyes yet, so I stare ahead, putting off the point when I will have to acknowledge her for a few more minutes.

My room resembles a rural B&B that's had a contemporary interior facelift. It has a functional en suite, window seat, and country views. Bob passes me forms to fill in that ask me to assess my self-risk and suicidal ideation. A nurse called Mary goes through my luggage. The usual suspects are confiscated, and this time my soap, shampoo, and conditioner are also removed.

The initiation talks take about 15 minutes, and then Bob, Mary, and Mum leave. I sit on the edge of my bed, listening to Mum and Dr Finch chatting in the hallway, realising that the fact that they have crossed paths means that Dr Finch is on her way to see me. Routines spin. My head fuzzes with all the mistakes I've made since arriving.

She knocks on the door, and I tense so hard I strain the muscles in my left leg. I cannot speak. The words will not come. She lets herself in, pulls the chair out from under my desk, and drags it so it is directly opposite me. Then she sits down.

'Hello.' She smiles.

'Hi,' I squeak.

'How are you?'

'Okay.'

'How are you really?'

'Bad.'

Silence.

'Do you need a minute?'

'Yes.'

Dr Finch folds her arms and sits quietly, patiently allowing me to finish the routines she knows are getting in the way of me talking to her. She is the only person who does that.

I love her.

I'm going to cry.

Except tears no longer come. When was the last time I cried? It's been months.

Stop! Focus. Finish the routines.

I tidy up the loose ends for a couple of minutes and then nod, signalling that I am done. I say done—I'm never really done when I only have two minutes, but I am done enough to attempt to engage in a conversation for a small window of time. Bursting point has been delayed.

'You're in a bit of a mess, aren't you?'

I nod.

'Okay. Let's try and disentangle a few things.'

A new regime is implemented. My medication is stabilised, with sleeping pills added to stop me staying up all night with my routines. I don't have to go to groups, but I do have to engage with my treatment. Dr Finch visits me three times a week, often staying for indefinite periods of time, while I perch on the edge of my bed and we work things out. These CBT sessions can go on for over two hours, as I confront whichever compulsions are the order of the day. Afterwards, I am so exhausted that I crawl under the covers and sleep. When I wake up, Mary will have brought me chocolate ice cream and put it in the kitchen fridge to make up for the meals I have missed.

Three other patients, Elizabeth, Catherine, and Sue, are on my ward. Catherine and Sue are in their forties, and Elizabeth is 65. They cluster together in the living room, happy to be herded and looked after by Mary. I keep my distance, sticking to my room and taking meals at my desk alone. When after four days I decide to go down for a meal in the dining room, it is a victory.

The dining room is vast and filled with lots of unused but immaculately laid tables. The hospital seems to have the capacity to house lots of patients, yet it has been almost empty since I arrived. I wonder if it is always that way. The four of us have lunch in a far corner with Mary. Mary tells us about the eating-disorder wards she used to work on, where patients who flatly refused food were held down and force-fed through tubes. We cannot believe it. In this day and age? How was it allowed?

'You don't understand,' says Mary softly. 'These people, they were killing themselves. We had to. We did it to save their lives. But it was too much. I ended up getting hurt a few times when people lashed out. That's why I work here. The pace is much slower.'

There is one critical problem with being here. Because I care about Dr Finch more than anyone, everything seems to be of life-changing importance. Even the slightest interaction with nurses, therapists, or other patients could be reported back to her, and so my lists expand and multiply by the second. I fear they are spying on me, waiting for me to do something bad so they can regale her with tales of my horrible nature:

BITCH

1. <u>M</u>ARY IN CORRIDOR: I heard Dr Finch talking to Mary in the corridor. I thought Mary said 'Did you just visit Princess Lily?' and was worried that they call me that because they think I am spoiled. Mary came in, and I asked her. She looked hurt and said 'I would never say that. I said 'Have you finished visiting Lily?' '

2. <u>P</u>HONE CHARGER: I wanted my phone charger, but the nurses wouldn't give me it. I said 'But you couldn't hang a dormouse with this.' This demonstrated an attitude problem and obnoxious nature.

BODILY FUNCTIONS:

1. <u>S</u>HOWER: Mary said 'I think you should have a shower, put your PJs on, and start relaxing so you sleep well tonight.' Was she trying to tell me that I smell and should shower more?

2. <u>P</u>ILLS: A male nurse I haven't seen before approached me in the corridor to give me my pills in a little paper cup. Then he took a step back. Did he do this because my breath smelled? Will he report to Dr Finch that I have a body odour problem?

3. <u>P</u>OO: It's been several days since I did a poo. I have been holding it in because I don't want to risk anyone knowing and telling Dr Finch. Tonight I had to go. Are there cameras in the bathroom, and does anyone know?

PERVERT:

1. <u>K</u>ISSY KISSY MUG: Bob had a mug in the nursing station

that said 'kissy kissy' on it and my eyes accidentally landed on it and stared at the words for a few seconds.

2. BRA AND PANTS: Mary came into my room, and I was in my bra and pants because I was about to have the shower she advised me to. Will she think I am a pervert who had been standing there waiting for someone to come in so I could expose myself?

VAIN:

1. NURSING STATION WINDOW: Caught reflection in the window when asking for charger.

2. COMPACT MIRROR: Another nurse called Elina came into my room, and my compact mirror was on the bedside table from earlier because at the moment I spend a lot of time checking there is nothing in my teeth. Did Elina see it and think I'm vain?

And on and on and on. I am on my seventh notebook. They are hidden in the drawer under the desk, with sweaters and T-shirts wrapped round them.

I wake up with a jolt, trying to shake off the sleeping-pill-induced fug. Something is wrong. I open my eyes to work out what is going on, but the room is filled with a blinding light. I force myself to focus.

Dr Finch is standing by the window, drawing my curtains like it's the most normal thing in the world.

I scramble to sit up straight. I am wearing my pyjamas. I haven't washed, brushed my teeth, or aired my room. What if the stench is unbearable? Dr Finch pulls the chair out from under my desk and sits opposite my bed. I am scrunched up in a ball against the headboard, looking at her in horror.

'What time is it?' I whisper.

'It's 10. What's wrong? Do you want me to give you a minute?'

'Yes!'

'Okay, no problem.'

She stands up and leaves my room, shutting the door quietly. I sit staring at the wall in shock, allowing the silence to settle for five seconds. Then I go into overdrive. Luckily, I requested my wash bag from Elina yesterday and she forgot to ask for it back, so at least I have some weapons. I shower, open windows, spray the room with perfume, and brush my teeth until they bleed.

It is bad enough when the nurses come in in the morning to check I am alive: if something is disgusting, they might notice and tell Dr Finch. But Dr Finch herself has just come within a of me in an unwashed state. I feel sick. It has been 10 minutes. She will be back soon. I grab my notepad and frantically start writing down the possible things she might have found repulsive and—

A knock on my door.

'Are you ready yet?'

'Uh . . .' I cannot kill any more time. She will think I am a weirdo with something to hide. 'Yeah . . . come in.'

The room reeks suspiciously of too much Dove deodourant and Miss Dior Cherie, but Dr Finch doesn't say anything. The session begins and goes on as normal, though admittedly I'm less cooperative than usual because I'm trying to compile the terrible events of the morning so far into something resembling a list. Forty-five minutes later, Dr Finch seems to decide she isn't getting much out of me, and she goes as swiftly as she came.

I am left sitting in bed in a cloud of routines. Then I find myself laughing, at first just a little, but it soon becomes uncontrollable, as if one minute I was a girl and the next I became I hyena. Because it seems so funny: I have spent so long dreaming of living with Dr Finch, but I can't even cope with her opening the curtains in the morning. Does the universe have a sense of humour?

Laughing at a routine is like flicking a switch on. It's not that everything suddenly changes, because brains don't seem to work that way. It is more like waking up and feeling excited because a thin layer of snow has covered the city, and now you are wondering what you should do with the day.

I am emboldened. I am going to make an effort. I am going to put myself in situations that involve talking to other people. I get up and go to the nursing station. Mary is sitting at her desk, updating the patient notes.

'Mary?'

She looks up.

'It's such a lovely day. Can you take us for a walk? Please?'

Mary checks her watch and looks out the window.

'Sure. In half an hour, okay? Ask the other ladies if they want to come.'

An hour later, Elizabeth, Catherine, Sue, and I are walking through a park with Bob and Mary. We are enveloped in acres and acres of green hills, and about 50 metres away, a mob of silky-haired deer straddling a hilltop stare us down.

'I'm going to see the deer!' I announce, running towards them.

Behind me, Mary yells out to be careful, but I can hear that she is laughing.

I get quite close and the deer still aren't running, but I slow down anyway, making it clear I mean no harm. I edge closer, until I am about five metres away. I stand, panting softly as I admire their shiny coats and the way their breath comes out their nostrils in clouds. The stag in the group pads towards me before coming to a halt and looking me up and down with purpose. The brown colours in his irises are in a constant state of movement; they are like burning haystacks, and they make me feel alive.

'Hey there,' I say.

I hear Bob calling me. I take a deep breath before turning around and running back to the group.

Mary is in a fit of giggles.

'Girl, you are so brave! You . . . just . . . I can't believe you just did that!'

Bob pulls a nervous grin. I feel bad now. I don't want to cause him stress.

'Sorry. I just . . . wanted to say hello!' I say.

'Okay. Just don't do that again.' He chuckles. 'You'll give me a heart attack!'

I add **R**UNNING TO DEER to my list in *SELFISH* as penance for causing him stress just so I could enjoy myself.

But I don't regret it.

Back at the hospital, I make a decision.

Exposing myself to the things I fear and learning to deal with them is the only way forward. It's possible I needed to be an inpatient to protect me from myself, but now I need to go.

I log on to my laptop and send an e-mail to my old employer at the nursery. I tell her that things didn't work out for me at university, and that I've left.

I say that I am available to work if they need anyone.

An hour later, I have a reply.

Sandra says she's sorry to hear my news, but delighted from her point of view. She tells me the nursery group happens to urgently need someone to start working mornings, at a different nursery to the one I was at before. Am I interested? Can I start tomorrow?

I stare at the e-mail, reading it over and over. My heart is racing. There's a knock on the door. Dr Finch comes in.

'What's up?' she asks.

'Don't get mad.'

'Have I ever?'

'No. But you might now. Here's the thing. I need to leave.'

'Why?'

'I contacted the nursery. I asked if there was a job for me. I didn't expect things to happen so suddenly, but they've got back and said there is a position. And I need to start tomorrow.'

Dr Finch laughs. It's not a mean laugh; it's a free laugh with a life of its own. It lasts for 10 seconds, and then she's back to normal.

'You never fail to surprise me. Ever.'

'I know you'll think this is crazy. And that it's like when I went off to college and was insisting I would just get better. But this isn't like that. I know it's not going to happen overnight. I'm only going to work mornings. It's going to be like proper exposure therapy. I'll take my treatment seriously. I'll have afternoons off, and I can come down from London for sessions with you. So you have to discharge me, please. Please.'

Dr Finch considers things for a few seconds. I feel sure she is going to say no.

'Okay. Why not? If it's what you want. You can come and see me two afternoons a week, and we can reevaluate things if it doesn't work out. At least you're not trying to leave the country.'

I am ecstatic. I want to jump up and down and dance.

'Thank you.' I grin. 'Genuinely. Thank you so much.'

Dr Finch gives me a small smile and smooths her skirt.

'If it's what you want,' she repeats.

Mum comes to get me in the Beetle. She's brought a guest.

'Ella!'

She helps me grab my suitcase and take it downstairs. Mum goes into the office to talk to the nurses about something. Outside on the driveway, Ella hoists the bag into the boot, and we both get in the back.

We are quiet for a while—there are no blueprints for little siblings who have to grow up five years in one day.

'Best sister ever,' she whispers.

26

Nursery

'Mum!' I hiss. 'Do you have to pull up so close to the nursery? Do you know how embarrassing it would be if anyone knew you were dropping me at work?'

I reel from the comments I have just made. They came out of nowhere. It takes a lot of energy to be a good person all the time and never show a trace of annoyance, and there are times, like just now, when my mask slips.

Mum looks surprised and hurt.

'Oh, sorry, darling. I didn't realise it was a problem. Of course, I can park around the corner. Sorry again.' She glances nervously at me, as if I am a newly discovered element that may react to things unpredictably.

'No, no, don't be. I didn't mean it to come out like that.'

I allow her to kiss me good-bye on the cheek. My skin burns where she pecks. I automatically add

CHEEK SMELL: Did my cheek smell?

CHEEK TASTE: Did she taste my skin where she touched with her lips? If so did it taste horrible?

to *BODILY FUNCTIONS*.

'Bye, love you,' I call, getting out and shutting the car door, checking that I don't leave any disgusting smudgy fingerprints on the paintwork.

I cross the road and buzz on the blue church door to be let in. Miss Rebecca and Miss Bianca, who share me as their teaching assistant, are busy setting up. Unlike the last nursery I worked in, this one rents space in a church hall, so we have to set up and pack away every morning. The two of them are hauling in sandpits, easels, tables, and tiny chairs from the shed where they are stored.

'Morning, Miss Lily!' they call.

'Morning!' I chirrup back.

This morning I am on Messy Tray, Role Play Area, and Snack.

Messy Tray and Role Play Area are specific areas of the classroom that the fascist Ofsted inspectors get very excited about, so they have to be set up perfectly in order to score top points should an inspector drop by.

I fill the Messy Tray with a jug of water mixed with blue food dye and glitter to make an ocean, before plopping in some plastic sea creatures (to enhance 'knowledge and understanding of the world'), foam alphabet numbers and letters (to enhance 'literary and numeracy'), and fishing rods (to improve 'motor skills'). I write what I have done in a file so that if Ofsted don't come today they can still look up the ways in which we helped the children develop intellectually and physically.

The Role Play Area changes once a week. We have had a farm, a shop, a Chinese restaurant, and a family home, and now we are setting up an accident and emergency department. I lay out mini stethoscopes, reflex hammers, bandages, and heart-rate monitors on a tiny consultation table, and then hang up doctors' and nurses' costumes under a sign that reads 'Hospital' in Korean. Ofsted also get very excited about multicultural signage. The children don't, as they can't read. We are missing a waiting area, and I find myself wondering if I should line 10 rows of chairs outside to prepare the children for a more realistic NHS experience.

'Everything okay, Lily?' calls Miss Rebecca from the other side of the hall. I realise I have been standing looking at the Role Play Area for a couple of minutes.

'Yep!' I call. I must prepare Snack.

It's my third day, and I haven't done Snack here before, but I assume it won't be any different from the last nursery. I go into the kitchen but can't find any apples. Nursery protocol is that apples should be cut wearing protective plastic gloves and aprons to stop the spread of germs.

I ask a senior teacher called Miss Louise where I can find apples, aprons, and gloves. She tells me the apples are in the shed, and that no one really bothers with the aprons or gloves.

'But, but . . . the regulations say we have to wear them,' I say, stammering slightly and hating myself for being a health and safety geek, but knowing that I won't let my bare hands touch, peel, and cut apples that will be eaten by actual children. I picture the 0.01 percent of germs that couldn't be washed off by the antibacterial soap crawling from my naked fingers deep into an apple segment, ready to be delivered into the innocent mouth of an unsuspecting child with a weak immune system . . .

'Well, you're right, we probably should be wearing them,' says Miss Louise. 'I think there's some in the back of the far-right cupboard.'

Protective clothing located, I open the shed door. The apples are lying in an open crate on the floor. There are animal droppings in the crate. I pick out some apples. They have teeth marks in them.

I run back to Miss Louise to tell her about the unfolding

disaster, but she is unfazed.

'Oh . . . okay. . . . Well, why don't you just give them an extra wash and keep peeling until you get through the bite marks?'

This is Ratgate.

'I'm not going to give the children apples that have been gnawed by rats. Those apples need to be thrown away. And from now on we need to keep apples inside, and not in the shed.'

'The apples can't stay inside,' says Miss Louise through gritted teeth. 'You know that we don't have the space. But okay, fine. We'll buy tight-seal plastic containers for the shed. In the meantime, you can take some money from the petty cash and get some biscuits for Snack today.'

The children arrive at nine. They swarm the classroom, destroying our meticulously arranged learning areas and reading corners in seconds, throwing the Plasticine, hiding in the bathroom, and painting the walls.

I sit them down to make paper-chain snakes for Chinese New Year. Alongside the interaction with Miss Louise, which is marked as a very red item in *RUDE*, the daily minutiae of normal routines are streaming in. At the moment I am debating whether adding paper chains to make the snakes longer and passing them off to parents as the children's work makes me a liar in breach of the Ofsted requirement for creativity to be child-led. I cannot disappear to the bathroom to write stuff down for the rest of the morning—we are understaffed as it is, and since I'm the shared assistant for two teachers, my leaving the room could result in chaos.

The last nursery I worked in felt more contained. But here the children are a year younger, and it's a jungle—every toddler for himself.

'Miss Lily!' screeches Miss Bianca, who is Japanese and bull-like, both in shape and personality. 'Stanley has done poo! Needs change!'

Here, I change nappies up to 10 times a morning, and each one is a dramatic exercise in doing absolutely nothing that could be construed as dodgy. Child-protection rules state we need to have two people present whenever a nappy is changed, but we don't have enough staff for that to be possible. We fill in forms recording the exact details of the change, and for each change there's a box where you need the signature of another staff member to prove they were there. Since 'we all have each other's backs here,' you're expected to ask someone to pretend they were there and sign, and then they return the favour for you later. I queried it yesterday, trying to sound offhand, but there isn't really a casual way to ask, 'Will anyone be supervising me when the children are in a potentially vulnerable situation?' Miss Bianca gave me a look that said *Only an actual paedophile asks that*.

Stanley plods over to me expectantly and stretches up his hand to be held as we walk to the baby-change station. The shit has leaked out the absorber pad and down his legs, and it takes a good 10 minutes to clean it up and change him into new trousers. Ten minutes is a suspiciously long time to spend changing a nappy by yourself. I add this fact to *PERVERT*. Unfortunately, his willy is caked in the turd, and I have to wipe it a few times to get it off. And that's when the unthinkable happens. Stanley gets an erection. It's tiny, the size of a little party sausage, but it's undeniably there. Oh, shit.

Later I find myself looking in the window of a local pet shop, before entering on impulse. I walk over to a stack of glass boxes, all of which contain various forms of slumbering tiny creatures in plastic hideouts lined with cotton wool.

In one, four or five white-and-ginger baby hamsters are huddled snoozing together. In the same container, a distinctly larger brown one crawls over to my finger at the glass.

'Why is this one so much bigger than the others?' I ask the guy behind the desk, who has long greasy hair and a lopsided mouth.

'Because we've sold all her siblings, but no one wanted her, because for some reason she was much bigger than the rest, so she's not so cute, you see? Those other little ones in the cage with her are a few weeks younger than her. They're selling well.'

Why would you put a fat hamster that you're struggling to sell in with a load of tiny cute ones? That's like dumping a hippo on the catwalk.

Bleakly, he adds, 'To be honest, it's looking like she might end up going to a lab . . .'

I have no idea if that is a realistic fate for an unsold hamster with a weight problem or a sales tactic. Either way, I'm buying.

I take Tubby into nursery every day in a travel box. The children love her.

They sit in a circle and I put her in the middle and she runs from child to child. Then they roll onto their fronts, and I let her crawl across their backs. Sometimes I put her in the top pocket of my smock and wander around with her peeking her little head out with her paws gripping the edge of the fabric. The children clap their hands together and yell in delight.

Tubby is not like the hamsters Ella had when she was little. Tubby is pretty much as tame as a dog. She remembers who you are and you can let her crawl around your room because she doesn't try to escape. One time I fell asleep with her in my bed and when I woke up a few hours later she was still there, curled up in the nook of my neck.

I sit with her in my room, letting her walk over my hands and up my arms. She is the only living thing who doesn't make me break into a sweat of routines. Is this what it's like for normal humans when they interact with other humans?

I put Tubby on a diet, but it doesn't help. In fact, she gets bigger. I feel she may have some sort of glandular problem, but others form their own theories.

'I sorry, but there is no way that is hamster,' belly-laughs Miss Bianca every morning. 'That is big ratty rat.'

I get home from work and take Tubby out of her travel box and place her carefully back in her cage. Then I collapse onto my bed and reach for my notebook to write down the words from the afternoon.

Dr Finch and I have agreed that I will not write down things that are of low importance. Words are of low importance if I can rationally understand that my behaviour wasn't bad. The idea is to move up gradually—next I will stop writing down the things of medium importance—until I don't write down anything at all.

Today, a girl called Annie asked if she could hold Tubby, and I said no, because I've given her three chances before and she always squeezes so tight that Tubby's little black eyes start bulging out of her head. Then I felt like a *BITCH*, but really, I've given her chances before, and what is so wrong with setting boundaries for a child and protecting an animal's welfare? So this is something I will not write down. There are other things that have happened today that I'm also able to dismiss and not put on this list, so I feel pleased.

Two-year-old Matteo has started simulating sex with a baby doll in the Role Play Area. It is witnessed by Miss Rebecca and me.

Miss Rebecca asks me what we should do, which is concerning, as I'm used to taking my orders from her. I say we should tell Miss Louise and take whatever appropriate action the guidelines say we should.

At first Miss Louise doesn't really believe us, and then she adopts a laissez-faire aren't-all-kids-a-bit-odd-though? attitude.

To be honest, I'm not sure. After a week of sleepless nights, I asked Mum about Stanley's erection. She said not to worry about it; that little boys often get erections. This was news to me.

'Matteo is foreign. Foreign people raise their children differently,' says Miss Louise. 'Maybe he sleeps in his parents' room? He's probably just copying what he's seen them doing at night. . . . I really don't think it's anything to worry about.'

Miss Rebecca protests that if Matteo is trying to tell us that he is being sexually abused, we have a moral responsibility and a duty of care to help.

'Well, let's wait and see if it happens again,' trills Miss Louise, breezing off to the other classroom with a cluster of child-led papier-mâché flowers for the 'Spring Has Sprung' board.

Miss Rebecca heads back to our classroom, her forehead still creased in concern. I stand where I am, wondering what to do, because I'm the only one who has been changing Matteo's nappy. What if he learned this behaviour from me?

Maybe I've been abusing Matteo, and I don't even remember it?

It happens several times more, and each time Miss Rebecca and I report back to Miss Louise.

On the fifth time, she realises she probably has to do something, and promises to take action.

I am waiting to be summoned for rigorous questioning; for fingers to be pointed; to stand in the dock as the accused. It will come out that we haven't been following protocol around here, and that I've been changing Matteo by myself.

'I remember she once asked if anyone will supervise her,' Miss Bianca will say. 'If only I realised then she was asking to make sure no one would catch her. It is so sad.'

My life is on hold as I stand braced for something awful to happen.

But the days turn to weeks, and no one so much as mentions my name.

It feels like I have gotten away with murder.

I sit in front of Dr Finch, crying, telling her that I got it wrong: all this time I was worried about doing something that would make someone mistakenly think I am a paedophile, while the truth is, I actually am one.

'This boy, Matteo,' levels Dr Finch. 'Do you actually remember abusing him?'

'No!' I say, sobbing.

'Then what makes you think you have?'

'Because I'm the only one who has been changing his nappy. . . . I need to quit my job to protect all the other children, and then I need to hand myself in to the police.'

'We know that people with OCD often become obsessed with the idea that they've committed a crime and they don't remember doing it. We know that worry that they've hurt someone becomes an intrusive thought that they fully believe in. Do you think maybe that might be what's happening here?'

'No.'

'Why?'

'Because it's too much of a coincidence, after what happened when I was younger, that suddenly there's this child who I've spent time with by myself and he's acting like he's been abused.'

'Maybe the coincidence is what's making it such a powerful fear?'

'No. No. No.'

'Do you think a real paedophile would get this stressed about having abused a child?'

'I don't know. It doesn't matter. I can't be around children.'

'Okay. I don't want to feed into this by giving you too much reassurance, but you know that that isn't the sort of thing you would do, and that children are very safe around you. I would be more than happy to let you babysit my children.'

Back at the nursery, I have seated the children from Miss Rebecca's class round the plastic table. They each have a few biscuits that we baked earlier this morning in front of them, along with some gold wrapping paper, stickers, and ribbons.

The biscuits are Mother's Day gifts. We want to involve the children in wrapping them up to enhance their 'knowledge and understanding of the world' and keep everything child-led, but it's quite fiddly, so essentially I'll wrap and they'll slap on a few stickers. Miss Rebecca told me to do this, so although it counts as lying, I will try not to write it down, because I can mark it as a less important item.

I dislike wrapping presents because I panic that I'll put

something inside that could get me in trouble when it gets opened. As I'm wrapping today, I worry that I've slotted a confessional note in with Matteo and Stanley's and cyanide in Phoebe's, and, weirdly, that I've eaten all the biscuits in Minnie's and just wrapped up air, crumbs, and a handwritten note saying 'yum ;).' I console myself that when the children have gone home, I'll unwrap the presents and check what is inside.

Minnie tells Izzie that her wrapped biscuits look nicer than Izzie's, and Izzie argues the point for a few sentences before she runs out of comebacks and starts to cry. She stretches her arms up to me for a cuddle and some comfort, but I don't trust myself to pick her up without hurting her. Without giving a cuddle, it takes over five minutes to calm her down. I add this to *INCOMPETENT*, which is my newest category, under the heading: COULD NOT CALM IZZIE QUICKLY.

Miss Bianca heads to the far corner of the room and shouts at Jamie and Tom for making a mess of the Messy Tray. This seems like a slightly unfair accusation, but since I am closer to that area than any other member of staff, and I didn't tell them not to splash, I also slot this failing in *INCOMPETENT*.

Later, when the children have gone home and we are packing away in exhausted silence, Miss Louise utters a blood-curdling shriek.

'Please tell me this is not what I think it is,' she wails, brandishing a pair of grown-up scissors in the air in one hand and clutching her chest with the other like a panto princess in shock. 'These were in children's scissor drawer!'

I absolutely know I would not be that careless. I absolutely know it wasn't me. I am absolutely sure.

Or am I?

No. I am not absolutely sure. I bet I did it on purpose, hoping that one of the children would find the scissors and hurt themselves.

My career in child care is not looking promising. I simply cannot foresee a future where every day is spent worrying so much about having hurt a child. I resolve to not work here past the end of the school year, and to find something different do with my life. But what?

27

Journalism

I used to want to be a journalist. So I apply to various magazines and papers, hoping that they will offer me an internship. At first I don't hear from any, and I worry that I will be unemployed for the foreseeable future.

But then a local magazine gets back to me, offering me two weeks of work experience over the summer.

I jump at it.

The guy I have been corresponding with about the placement is Doug. He peppered his e-mails with elaborate turns of phrase that were supposed to look casual but didn't and kept harping on about an interview he'd recently done with Vince Cable. When I imagined him behind the keyboard, I saw a balding, slightly plump 50-year-old man, probably wearing a knitted tank top.

But Doug, who meets me in the entrance hall, is not 50. Doug is about 25, has surfer-blond hair, electric-blue eyes, and skinny jeans. He is, quite frankly, probably the most attractive person I've ever seen. He introduces himself and leads me upstairs to 'meet the team.'

It is not glamorous. The software is stuck somewhere in 2005; the blinds don't work and are missing half of their slats; the carpet, I am told almost immediately, comes from a skip. But there is something warming about it anyway: the promise of sparky, creative people, hammering stories out at their computers; photoshopping and designing page layouts and constantly popping out for cigarette breaks.

Which is why it is all the more aggravating that my head won't shut up.

My first task is to research a piece about local vintage experiences. Doug tells me to trawl the web for the best way to go retro in Surrey. It is cheesy and old hat, but it's also the sort of piece I know I can do. It's essentially a Google-and-bullshit job; I just can't get to the bit where I open Google.

Every interaction so far has been like watching a vase shatter into hundreds of tiny pieces that can't all be picked up; everything I do sets off a chain reaction of words. And I can't keep going to the bathroom to write them in my notebook, because I don't want to be remembered as the nervous intern with the shits.

So I will do what I did at nursery. I will wait until lunch, when I can go somewhere private for a scribble fest. In the meantime, I will hold the words in my head. But I'm terrified I'll forget some. What is the point of writing a good piece, if I do awful things that I can't remember (but which everyone else can)?

It takes about 45 minutes to identify the words I need to hold, during which time I continuously type, delete, and retype the ultimately crap sentence 'There are many ways to go vintage in Surrey,' hoping I look so busy that no one will notice my private chaos.

I use a ballpoint pen to write down the first letters of words on my hand so I have some cues for later. I haven't done this since I was in the hospital. This is a bad thing to start doing. But I want this work experience to go perfectly, so everything has to be remembered.

'Does everything have to go perfectly?' Dr Finch says loudly, as though she is in the room. 'Is perfection ever truly attainable? And, say it were, would it be desirable?'

'We do have notepads, you know! We're shabby, but we're not that shabby!' calls Doug from his desk.

Shit.

Brigitte, the French production manager who has been sitting behind me, spins around.

'Ooh la la!' she exclaims. 'Your hands are so red! You should not be writing on them! They must be agony! Here, have some hand cream.'

'Thanks.' I blush. 'They're, uh, they're a bit sensitive, yes. Thank you,' I say, massaging in the cream.

Sensitive?

Liar.
Liar.
Liar.

I turn back to the computer. The seven words generated from that interaction demand my full attention. I spend a couple of minutes sorting them before opening Google, knowing that I urgently need to start going vintage in Surrey.

I lift my hands, poised to type.

Any second now I will start typing.

Any second.

But I can't.

I am gripped by the sudden fear that I'm about to start Googling lewd things.

Vintage cock rings.
Retro dildos.

Reclaimed crotchless pants.
Secondhand XXX videos.

This is too much.

'I need a brew,' announces Doug to the room. 'Lily, do you want to help me do the tea run? I can show you where everything is.'

'Uh . . . Yeah, sure.' I smile.

Doug rounds the room, sweeping mugs off people's desks and putting them on a grimy silver tray.

'You can make the tea,' he says. 'I'll do the coffees. Tea bags there, hot water there, milk in the fridge. Sugar in that pot.'

I have four teas to make, two of which must be sweet. I worry that instead of spooning sugar into them, I've pulled some rat poison from my pockets and sprinkled it in. There is a toilet coming off the kitchen. This is unhygienic. I convince myself that I've quickly whizzed in there when Doug's back was turned and pissed in the mugs.

People cannot drink these teas. It's not going to happen. I tip three of them down the sink, quickly, before Doug can stop me (I'm not concerned about mine being contaminated, because you can't go to prison for poisoning yourself, especially if you're dead).

'Why would you—'

'Doug,' I say, preparing to fill up the *IDIOT* category, 'I don't think I've made the teas how they wanted them. Can you make them, and I'll watch so I get it right next time?'

Doug raises an eyebrow and laughs.

'It's tea, not rocket science!'

Great. Sexy work guy now thinks I'm a total moron. I resolve to get out of all future tea making. I don't care if it's a rite of work-experience passage. No one is going to die on my watch.

Bill, the editor-in-chief, calls me into his office.

I sit in the swivel chair across from his desk and try to keep as still as possible to minimise wrongdoing.

'I'm very impressed with your vintage piece,' says Bill. 'I think we'll run it next month.'

'Thank you.' I try to smile the right amount—enough for him to know I am pleased by the compliment, but not so much that I look deranged. I do not tell him, or anyone, that I wrote the vintage piece at home, as I did everything else I was set this week. Away from prying eyes, with all lists in order and only Tubby for company.

The next comment takes me off guard.

'Would you like a job?'

'I . . . uh . . . Yes! I would love a job!'

Idiot.

Idiot.

Idiot.

'How are you with websites?'

'I'm not great. But I could learn.'

The vintage piece needs images to go with it. I manage to get some beautiful sketches of 1960s outfits on mannequins from the owner of a nearby shop I'm featuring. They're perfect—but they're original hard copies, and Brigitte says we need digital versions or they can't be laid out on the page.

The sketches are too big for our scanner, which means I need to go to the photocopy shop and get them scanned there. Brigitte says it's close—if I get the bus, I can be there and back in less than an hour. I place the sketches in the giant plastic folder they arrived in and set off.

The flood starts before I'm even out the door. The things I've done wrong this morning take centre stage, and I'm so engrossed in them that it takes me by surprise when I find that I have arrived and walked into the shop. A man comes out from behind the counter and shows me what to do. Each page gets scanned and whizzed onto Brigitte's memory stick. I pay and leave. Simple. Job done. But—

I still have to sort out all the stuff from this morning. Dazed, I get on the bus and try to smooth it out. After 30 minutes I've not gotten anywhere with it. And wait—none of this looks familiar. Where am I? I ask the driver. He says I've taken the bus in the wrong direction. So off I get, panicking that it's now going to have taken me longer than Brigitte said. Never mind, I'll go back in the other direction, and while I'm doing that I'll sort the stuff in my head out. Wait, where am I now? I've taken the wrong bus entirely. Oh shit, oh shit, shit, *shit*. I'm going to be so late. I'm going to ruin everything. I get off the bus and look at the bus map. My lists are fizzing, demanding proper attention. Okay, I'll stand here and sort them out, then I can concentrate properly. But that just makes me lose another 10 minutes, and I'm no closer to fixing them. I look at the bus map again.

There's no space in my head for it. It might as well be in Spanish.

I'm going to run, I'll just keep running, one foot in front of the other, until the list goes away and—

I don't want you to have to deal with this on your own, said Mum. *I want to help you, but you need to let me in.*

My hands do my thinking for me. I take my mobile out my pocket and press the green call button. Mum answers after a few rings.

'Hello?' The line is funny—echoey, like she's in a big cave. I hear the rhythmic plod of a distant ball going back and forth—the squeak of trainers on a vinyl indoor court.

'Help me!' I wail. 'I've got onto two wrong buses and I'm late and I'm going to fuck it all up! Please come and get me and help me find my way back to the office!'

'Darling, I'm at my tennis lesson. Slow down, what happened?'

I try to explain, but I'm finding it hard to breathe.

'Okay,' she says. 'I'm coming! I'm in Fulham, though. I may take a little while. Just stay calm. Stay calm!'

I see a National Health Service hospital up ahead. I find myself walking through the doors and taking a seat on a plastic chair in the waiting room. I text Mum and let her know where I am.

My phone is ringing. It's Mum.

'I'm here!' she says. 'Come outside! I'm just on the left.'

There she is sitting in the silver Beetle—her accomplice. I get in next to her. She's in full tennis whites—a sweatband round her head, sporting a spaghetti top and a tiny Adidas tennis skirt.

'Did you really want to go to hospital?' she asks.

'I just didn't know what to do. I was scared.'

'Do you want to go back to work?'

'I think so.'

'Okay!' she hammers the address into the satnav and starts to weave through traffic.

It doesn't take very long.

'Darling, it was pretty much round the corner!'

She parks on the opposite street, and I feel my courage fail me. I feel extra stupid, knowing how close we were.

'I can't go in,' I say.

'You can! It won't be as bad as you think, I know it.'

'You go!' I'm five years old again, seeing the world from behind the pillar of a parent's leg. 'You have to! Explain to them that I'm really sorry, but I can't do it.'

'Me? Like *this*?' She gestures to her outfit.

As I see her stand up to go, the ridiculousness of how it's going to look hits me full throttle.

'I'm Lily's mum,' she'll say, as the whole office turns to gawp at her perfectly bronzed legs. 'I was just playing a spot of tennis when I received a call from my distressed daughter, to tell me that she couldn't work out how to read a bus map . . .'

'Okay, wait! Don't go. I can do it.'

'Good,' she says, sitting back down. 'I wasn't looking forward to that. Go—don't waste any more time. You'll be fine. I believe in you!'

I run out the car and only look back once. My mum, my one-woman fan club, is cheering me on.

Back on the editorial floor, there is no trouble awaiting me. Just a few colleagues, who think it's hilarious when they find out that I got so lost.

Mum was right. I'd swelled up a storm that only I could see.

Here's to the strong ones. Here's to the ones who never give up.

Dad and his girlfriend Charlotte—blonde, yoga teacher, super hot—have moved to Oxford to do up a vicarage and start a family.

Ella and I are visiting them for the weekend.

'We need to get in the car,' says Dad on Saturday morning

when we've finished catching up over brunch and I have told him about the job offer. 'We're going on a trip.'

The four of us pile into the Porsche Cayenne. Charlotte, who is six months pregnant, sits in the front, absent-mindedly stroking the neatest bump known to womankind.

We glide down country lanes before joining the motorway, headed towards our mystery location. We exit in Reading, cruising down suburban streets, before pulling up at a row of ugly bungalows.

'What do you want for your twentieth birthday?' Dad said.

'A puppy!' I laughed, not really thinking anyone would deem me responsible enough.

Two months ago I turned 20. I know where we are.

'Dog breeders always live in the weirdest places,' confirms Dad.

'Oh my god!' I grin. I flash back to all those years ago, when we picked Tuffy up in similarly mysterious circumstances. Dad has always loved surprises.

We get out of the car, and Dad rings the bell. I see shadows moving towards us through the glass, and hear hurried footsteps getting closer. A stocky man in a polo shirt with a big pearly-white smile and a tanned face opens the door.

'Hi! I'm Bert! You must be here to see the puppies! We only have two left now! Breeding runs in my family, we've been doing it for generations!' says Bert. He is one of those people who end every sentence on a high note. I feel like I've just walked onto the set of a low-budget advert.

'Please, come in!'

The four of us follow Bert through the kitchen and into a utility room, where two balls of white fluff are curled up at the back of a newspaper-lined cage. Their mum snoozes in a basket at the other end of the room.

'You can pick whichever one you like!' says Bert, opening the cage door.

I don't want to pick a dog. Showing such brazen favouritism will invariably end up as a very red item in multiple categories.

'Aww, that feels kinda unfair!' I say, trying to keep it light and airy, while disliking myself for adding an Americanised twang to the word *kinda*, and joining Bert by soaring up on the word *unfair*. 'I'm sure neither of them will be offended!' comforts Bert awkwardly.

'I'll just take whichever one comes to me first,' I say, getting down on my knees in front of the open cage.

The slightly larger puppy, who has been looking us up and down since we walked in, pads out of the cage and tries to scramble onto my lap. He slips down the first two times, before giving me a cute, wide-eyed look that seems to say *This is the part where you help me*, so I scoop him up. He stares up at me triumphantly, little black nose twitching, tail wagging on my thigh. He looks like a Rocky.

'You can't take him upstairs!' Mum said. 'Oh my god. What if he has an accident?'

'Then I'll clean it up.'

'But you hate dirt. Surely dog pee in your room is your worst nightmare?'

'It's puppy pee. It doesn't feel that bad. It's like when Ella and I used to share a bath and Ella would pee in it and I would squeal and you told me not to worry because baby pee is magic healing water. 'They filter Evian through babies' bladders,' you said. Do you remember that? Well, now I sort of have the same positive feeling towards puppy pee.'

'You are a nutter!' Mum laughs. She clasps her hand to her mouth.

I put Rocky at the bottom of the staircase, but the first step is twice his height. He stares from me to the step and then back to me, sticking his pink tongue out a little in concentration. Then I realise he probably hasn't seen a staircase before. What must it be like to not know what a step is? I'd love to go back to that level of development. I'd love to learn everything all over again, but learn it right this time. I'd love to return my brain to factory settings.

I pop Rocky on my bed. I start checking things so that I can sit down and snuggle with him. I flick all the plug and light switches on off, on off, on off, and open and shut the blinds nine times. Rocky has sat up and is looking at me. He tilts his head at me, like he is wondering what the hell I am doing. He yaps once, high-pitched and deliberately. I would never normally do my routines in front of anyone, but I didn't count Rocky because I thought he would have no idea what I was doing. But he has noticed that something isn't quite right.

Even a puppy knows what I'm doing is odd.

I now feel awkward about carrying on.

I sit down on the bed and pick him up, stroking the velvety soft arch between his eyes. He relaxes; his eyelids droop.

'What do you think, Rocky? Should I take the job?'

He stretches his tongue out lazily and licks my palm. Then he falls asleep. I start telling myself that if he opens his eyes when I ask the question again, then it means I should take the job and that it will go well for me. Then I remember that I am not supposed to engage in magical thinking, and that it is not sensible to ask a puppy for advice.

The euphoria of the job offer dazzles less now that a couple of days have passed. I think I should probably be realistic and tell Bill that I might be able to take the job in a few months. But what reason am I going to give? Personal reasons? Having 'personal reasons' always makes you sound unemployable.

And will the job still be there?

I toy with the idea of deciding that I'm just going to do it anyway and get better somehow, but then I remember the times that has gone wrong before.

'I know you really don't want to,' says Mum after dinner. 'But why don't you try going to a support group? I'm not saying Dr Finch can't help you. I think she helps, but trying something else really can't hurt. Would you try it? For me?'

28

Rocky

I'm standing outside the support group room with my mum.

I peek in through the door's glass window. I see a huge circle of people sitting on plastic chairs.

'I've changed my mind, Mum. I don't want to go.'

'Come on, we've come all this way—just go in for a little bit and see how you find it. I'll be right by you.'

'I don't want to. I really, really don't want to.'

I peek in again. I see a woman with long brown hair talking, but I can't hear what she is saying. She is making lots of gestures.

Mum opens the door and pushes me in. I let out a loud squeak. About 30 heads turn to look at me.

'Welcome! Have a seat,' says a man sitting in the corner of the room. 'We're doing introductions. So you just have to say your name, your experience of OCD, and how your week has been. And you're welcome to pass if you would prefer not to say anything.'

I sit next to Mum on the other side of the circle. Each person speaks for a minute or two. I pass when it gets to me, but Mum makes up for that.

'This is Lily, and I'm her mum. It's our first time at a support group. Lily doesn't really want to be here, but I'm hoping that it will be helpful for her. I'm here because I want to learn more about OCD and how I can help Lily. Hello, everyone!'

She gives a little wave.

'Welcome, both of you,' says the man again. He actually does sound quite welcoming.

It's odd, because I always assumed that if I met a group of people with OCD, they'd all be sitting on newspapers to avoid contamination with the chairs, wearing gloves and perhaps surgical masks, tapping things repetitively.

But everyone here looks normal, and only a few of them have contamination fears.

I also thought there would be no point going to a group like this, because no one would have similar obsessions to me, but it seems that was wrong too.

'I always wanted to be a teacher, which I am,' says the girl opposite me. 'But I ended up teaching adults, because I'm scared I'll harm children if I'm around them.'

'I've had a really bad week because I feel like these thoughts are never going to stop,' says one guy.

Another says, 'My OCD centres on preventing harm. So if I see anything in the street that could be hazardous, like glass or whatever, I have to do something about it. I'm always looking out for things that could cause harm so I can remove them. And I have some contamination problems. But I've had a really good week. I feel like I'm having a breakthrough with my CBT.'

'My OCD also revolves around stopping bad things happening,' says someone else. 'Particularly to animals. Last week I saw a frog on the pavement so I tried to move him to a grassy knoll so he wouldn't get trodden on.'

'I do that!' chips in a guy across the room. 'I pick up snails and slugs from the pavement and rehome them. I also retrace my steps to make sure I haven't trodden on one.'

'Anyway, so I pick this frog up, yeah—and he jumps out of my hand, right into the road. And then bam, right in front of me—squashed by a car.'

There's a collective intake of breath as the group acknowledges the psychological implications of sod's law conspiring against the frog Samaritan.

'Yeah,' he adds. 'I was pretty upset.'

Halfway through, people talk to each other during a 15-minute break. The man who welcomed us comes over to introduce himself as Thomas and asks how I am doing.

For the second half he calls for quiet.

Conversations fade out, and people who have moved around scurry back to their seats. Across the room, the woman who said that she crochets to keep herself focused on something other than her thoughts goes back to making an orange scarf.

'Our discussion topic today is guilt, how it affects us, and what we can do to overcome it.'

There's a collective murmur of approval at the choice of topic.

'Oh god, don't even get me started on guilt!' says someone. 'I've got enough guilt on me to go round the whole of the UK prison system!'

Everyone laughs.

I feel like I have come home.

Later I lie in bed, feeling more comforted than I can ever remember feeling. There are people like me. Others out there who spend their days caught in the peaks and troughs of endless thought.

I am not a freak.

I roll over and put my arm around Rocky, who is curled up next to me. I breathe in the soft talcum-powder smell of his fur and listen to him snoring gently. I'm so glad I'm not alone anymore.

Since Rocky has been sleeping up here, I've stopped opening and shutting drawers and wardrobes to make sure nothing is inside, and stopped checking behind the curtains and under the bed.

Rocky makes the room feel okay. And I don't like to check stuff in front of him. If I do, he tilts his head to one side and gives me such a strange look that I feel stupid—which is helpful. It's good to be reminded how silly the things I do are, and because he's a dog, I don't resent him the way I would if a human was bleating at me to 'just stop doing it.'

I remember what Dr Finch said: 'Your routines feed off isolation.'

I can't sit at home all day, waiting for the help to come. That's only going to make it worse. But I also can't pretend there's nothing wrong; that only makes me crash eventually.

And that's when the answer I have been looking for suddenly arrives, like a gift: so simple, so pure, it's amazing I didn't think of it before.

I'll be honest.

I arrange to meet Bill in his office at 10.00am on Monday morning, but it's 10.15, and he's still in a meeting.

I sit outside, sipping nervously on a cup of tea Doug has made me and trying to engage with what he is chatting to me about. Brigitte and her production assistant Nel come and join the conversation. Everyone here is nice. They coo over me, laughing about how if I take the job, I will be the new office baby.

'I can't believe you're only 20! The youngest person gets to decorate the Christmas tree,' says Nel. 'So your luck's in this year!'

Bill finally calls me in at 10.45. I take a seat opposite him. Deep breath.

'Have you thought about my offer?'

'Yes,' I say. 'I've thought about it a lot. I would very much like to take the job. Thank you so much for offering me it.'

'Great! When can you start?'

'I can start as soon as you like. There's just . . . There's just one thing . . .'

'Oh yes?'

'I have OCD. And I'm trying to beat it at the moment. So I would need one afternoon a week off so I can see my doctor. And it's possible that sometimes, if it's going really badly, I might miss some work. I realise I've just made myself sound totally unemployable. But it's either tell you and take the job, or not take the job at all, because I've tried covering it up before, and it always ends badly. And I . . . I really, really want to take this job. So I thought I'd just put it out there and see if you could still take me on.'

Shut up now, shut up.

I prepare for Bill to give one of three standard responses:

'Oh, I'm also so OCD!'

'Aren't we all a bit OCD?'

'You can come and clean my house!'

What he says next takes me by surprise.

'What's OCD?' He looks a little embarrassed. 'I mean, sorry, I know I should know, but I don't.'

'No, don't worry at all. Well it stands for obsessive-compulsive disorder. So people who have it obsess over something, like a thought, or a worry, and then they do a compulsion to make that thing go away. And they get into a cycle where they can't stop doing those compulsions.

'So I . . . I worry a lot about all the actions I do, like how I say stuff, and whether it looked funny when I did something, or whether something about me appeared disgusting, and then I have to write it down and think about it a lot to make it go away. I fill up endless notebooks making lists of everyday stuff that other people don't think about. It takes up hours of every day. I'm also quite scared of dirt, so I wash my hands a lot. That's probably more what OCD is known for.'

The only person I tell this to is Dr Finch. I suddenly feel vulnerable and idiotic. Why am I telling a future boss about it?

'I know it sounds silly,' I add hastily.

'It doesn't sound silly, it sounds hellish!'

Oh. Sympathy. That's nice. I feel a little bolder.

'It is quite. Other people have different obsessions and compulsions, and it covers a huge range of things, because you can pretty much obsess over anything, so it's quite hard to explain. But anyway . . . I . . . I totally understand if you think it's not going to be possible to take me on.'

This is not a lie; I would totally understand. If I were organising a workforce, I wouldn't employ my brain.

'No, it's not a problem. I'm still very happy to offer you the job. Thank you for telling me about it. It's, er, it's good to be open about these things.' He pulls a sheepish grin, and I get the feeling that even though mental health is still the elephant in this room, the room is trying to accommodate the elephant, which is more than I expected.

'So you've been at the new job this morning?' asks Dr Finch, my folder on her lap, pen poised, ready to document this groundbreaking new development.

'And you decided to tell them about your OCD, didn't you? How did they take it?'

'Yes, I told them. They've been really great. My boss says I can take one afternoon off a week to see you. I go for lunch with two of my colleagues, Doug and Brigitte, every day at the café down the road. They asked me about the afternoon I'm taking off and I told them a bit about my OCD and they were really nice about it. I feel good.'

That was the easy part. Now for the hard bit.

'I think you maybe have some idea of how I feel about you,' I say in a rush. The words hang in the air, undoable, dangerously precluding their end.

'It is a feeling I wish I didn't have. It is a feeling that I think has sometimes got in the way of my treatment, because it makes me focus on perfecting my lists when I'm around you, rather than letting you show me how to fight them. It is a feeling that makes it painful to be in your presence, and for that reason, I need to get better as soon as possible, so that I can stop seeing you. Can we do that?'

'Yes,' says Dr Finch. 'Yes, we can.'

'Hi, I'm Lily, and I've had OCD since I can remember.'

I look around the group. People are nodding and smiling. Katie, who I've been to dinner with a few times and is becoming a good friend, grins and waves.

'It mainly centres on needing to record any actions that could be seen as bad and then justifying why what I did wasn't bad, or if it was bad, remembering why it was bad. My week has been quite good, actually. I've managed to start a new job. And I told my boss about my OCD, and he was unexpectedly supportive.'

The group seems genuinely pleased to hear this. Round the circle, others take their turn to do their introductions.

'I've had a good week,' says a woman called Sheila. 'I've discovered that what really helps me is putting off my compulsions. I tell myself I'll do it in five minutes, or maybe 10, and I keep saying that, and then eventually I realise the urge to do it has passed, and I don't need to do it anymore. It works really well for me.'

A chorus of other people say that they've found doing the same thing helpful.

I think about this strategy. Although it seems like I put my routines off, as I don't fully assess them until I'm by myself, I'm always concentrating on going over them in my head so I don't forget them. What if I tried to properly put them off? Could it work for me too?

The next day at the office, I adopt the mantra 'Work now, worry later.' Words come into my head, and I tell myself that I will give them my attention later. From an anxiety perspective, I don't feel the sheer terror that comes when I apply the orthodox CBT strategy of saying I will resist all routines.

Putting off the routines that arose in the first 10 minutes of work when everyone was chatting and saying hello means that, for the first time in my two weeks here, I've managed to get some work done before 10.00am.

I am inputting local news stories into our online publishing software. A missing boy, aged 14; a new celebrity moving to the area; the verdict of a trial of a local sex offender.

At this point, I'd normally spend a couple of hours thoroughly checking through the articles to see that I haven't chucked in some rogue concluding line like 'thanks for reading folks. FYI, I'm also a sex offender,' or 'Just so you know, the missing child is actually in my cellar.'

Today, I only check through for standard spelling and grammar, and then hit the Publish button. I tell myself it's okay, because I can check through them later.

The articles go live. I copy the links from our website and paste them into our Twitter accounts, typing the corresponding headlines into the tweet. I don't read the tweet over and over to check I'm not about to publish 'Saggy Granny Tits Are Coming to Surrey' or something similarly career-ending.

Bill calls me into his office for a chat about website stats. He is pleased with my progress. We chat for about 45 minutes. I go back to my desk. I want to check, but I tell myself I can do it later.

Brigitte calls me over to ask what I think of one of her page layouts. I pop out for a cigarette.

Later, later, I say.

I sit down and do some reading about a local pub for an article I might write on best cosy winter hangouts.

Later, later.

I go for lunch. I laugh with Brigitte about something stupid her cat has done.

Later, later.

I get back to my desk, take a phone call from an aggrieved local who wants to see more online coverage about golf. I've put down the phone and prepared to tell myself that I'll think about my lists in another five minutes, when I realise they are no longer causing me fear.

They are just a string of irrelevant actions that happened in the last few hours, and I don't need to change them.

29

The Truth

I am sitting in a bar opposite a man called Dean. He looks older than me, but not too old: maybe late thirties.

There's something about him I like. He is funny, but he doesn't seem to know it. I have 10 items on my list at present.

'What would you like to drink?' he asks.

I want these routines to stop. Just once, I want to enjoy the company of another human. I know I'm not supposed to drink to make it stop, but there's no denying it helps. No one need know.

'Wine,' I say.

We order glasses of chardonnay. Dean sips his at neat, regular intervals, seemingly at ease with the whole situation, and I pretend to be.

We talk about his life, we talk about mine. He holds my hand across the table, and I break my rule about not kissing on first dates. He is the sort of person with whom a couple of hours feels like not very much time at all, and also, he has nice eyes. I drink more wine. At around midnight, Dean decides I have had too much to drink. I am insisting I can get the Tube back. Dean initially agrees, but I don't quite pull off my sober strut down the stairs to Bond Street underground.

'No, okay, look, just come back with me, my car is round the corner. You need to sober up,' he says. 'Then I'm going to get you a taxi back.'

For some reason, this sounds like a great idea.

I remember the car ride in bits. I remember making Dean pull over outside a Lebanese restaurant so I can pee. I remember singing along to the radio. I remember getting to his flat and feeling sick. I remember sitting on the sofa with him. For how long? Twenty minutes? An hour? I remember thinking he really must be a very nice man, since he doesn't try to take advantage, or even touch me. I remember telling him that if I can't be perfect, I don't want to exist. I remember him calling me a taxi, good as his word, and making me promise to text him when I get home safely.

'Lily! You need to get up for work!' My mum is screeching up the stairs.

I burrow under the duvet, trying to shut out the day and return to the point on my list last night where I started forgetting things. I need to see what, if anything, I can retrieve. I know that I've accumulated Blank Time again, which is always a bad thing.

The easy option would be not to see Dean again, because then I don't have to think about the number of interactions that are unaccounted for. In fact, that would probably be the sensible option, given that he's too old for me and has teenage children. But actually, it doesn't even matter.

I think I suitably disgraced myself last night.

I doubt he will text. I'm wrong.

I have just arrived at Dean's flat. We are going to spend Saturday together, because, for some reason, he has decided he wants to see me again.

At my feet, Rocky is yapping and chasing his tail like an idiot.

'I think we should get this one to the park!' I say, adding **B**OSSY ABOUT ROCKY to *RUDE*, because you shouldn't tell someone what to do when they invite you to their home. But Dean doesn't seem offended. He clips on Rocky's lead with male efficiency, and away we go to Regent's Park.

Dean tries to take my hand twice. This is probably my fault for letting him hold my hand on our first date—the alcohol made me care less about physical contact. But in today's sober state, I am keen not to do anything disgusting.

I dodge him twice successfully, but he makes it the third time. I add **C**LAMMY HANDS as a red item to *BODILY FUNCTIONS*. The worst part about something like having clammy hands is that it is a real and disgusting problem, and all the CBT in the world won't make it go away.

I let Rocky off the lead, but he trots along between us, underneath the arch of our hands, on his best behaviour.

Dean laughs. 'He's so cute! He's walking between us like a little child!' I start to worry fervently that Dean might think I've trained Rocky to walk like this to convince him how nice it would be if we had children of our own, even though we've only met twice.

I add **M**ANIPULATIVE DOG OWNER to *BITCH*.

Halfway through lunch at a pub down the road from Dean's house on our fifth date, he asks me what's wrong.

The truth is, nothing is especially wrong; it's just I'm five minutes behind current time, analysing a sexual innuendo I may or may not have made.

I adopt my honesty-is-the-best-policy approach.

'I'm sorry,' I say. 'The truth is, I have OCD.'

He doesn't say anything stupid; he just lets me explain how it is. I tell him the more I care about someone, the more I care what I do around them. I tell him that every time I see him, I care about him more . . .

'And so your routines are getting worse?' he finishes.

'Yes. Exactly.'

'Okay,' he says, pausing, wiping the corners of his mouth with his napkin and placing it on his lap.

'So you have a choice. You can either continue seeing me and just accept that I love being around you and there's no need to do your routines, or you can do what you're doing, and eventually, a few weeks or a few months from now, or however long it takes, you'll end this yourself because it will get to the stage where you can't take it anymore.'

I could emphatically deny this, but the truth is, I have been thinking maybe I should end it while it's still a nice little romance I can remember fondly, before it gets totally destroyed by endless documentation.

'Why don't you just treat this whole thing like an experiment?' says Dean. 'Don't do any routines around me. Then, three months from now, if you can't bear to be with me because there's too much stuff you haven't accounted for, just walk away and start a new relationship with someone else and you can go back to what you were doing before, and know that all your interactions were perfect. But if, three months from now, you realise that you didn't need to do them after all, and that you're happy, then stay.'

It's brutal. It's radical. It includes a get-out-of-jail-free card. I like it.

This is how the next months go. I go to work, where I put off my routines until I don't fear them so much, and I get to a stage where I write down only the very red stuff. I start to have more of a personality, which is ironic, because I always thought it was my lists that meant I knew who I was.

The experiment is both terrifying and liberating. I become more and more able to dismiss the words that come up around Dean by thinking of the whole thing as a giant game of exposure therapy. I go to his place pretty much every night, because, I reason, I should get as much time in with him as possible before the three months are up.

But why do the three months have to be up? What if I make this experiment my life? It has to be better than what came before. And if this really is just a giant exposure where you do something scary to test your previously held theory about something, then the results are pretty clear: I didn't do my lists around someone. That person did not start to think I was a bad person and did not want to get away from me. Therefore, I do not need to do lists to stop being seen as a bad person.

Two weeks ago, Dr Finch came back to an idea we had spoken about when I first saw her.

'Your routines are like insurance where the premium is too high. Imagine if I paid so much insurance on my house that I ended up paying more than the actual value of the house. Well, that's what you do. You try to insure your life through doing endless routines, but the cost of that OCD insurance is too high, because you end up ruining the life you do have.

'Is it better,' she asked, 'to do all these routines so you can feel sure you're in control of everything you might possibly have done wrong, but end up miserable—or is it better to take the risk of letting some stuff go, but end up happy?'

I know which one I would have chosen before, and it's not what I would choose today. I choose to take a risk in the pursuit of feeling human. Whenever I do come back to my house from Dean's, if Ella is home from school, then I open my arms and pull her into a big cuddle. Every time I do it, I get a little less scared that I will harm her, and last week, when her curls tickled my cheeks and her arms twisted around my back, I felt nothing more than that I was one half of something hugging the other.

She doesn't know this is our last session.

We are 45 minutes through, and I still haven't told her. We have talked about how much better I am. We have talked about how I can keep the improvements going. We have talked about how to avoid relapsing. We have talked and talked, endless toing and froing for three years, and now here we are. Fifteen minutes left to know each other.

'I'm not coming back,' I say, waiting for the room to cave in on me.

It doesn't.

'And it's not like before. This is it. I'm better than I've ever been, and it's mostly thanks to you. And I . . . I won't be coming here again.'

Dr Finch doesn't do anything for a few seconds, which is unlike her.

'Okay,' she finally says, slightly higher than normal, with a smile that starts to wobble, like her face is going to crack. 'I don't know what you've done to me!' Her eyes brim with a few disobedient tears, which roll down her cheeks. 'I don't do this.' She wipes them fiercely, laughing at herself.

'I have—' Her voice catches, and she starts again, almost

whispering this time. 'I have known you for a long time.'

And because there is nothing more to say, we walk down the stairs and into the car park. I get into the taxi, which takes me to the station, where I board an empty train back to London.

I stare out the window at the trees whizzing by, wondering which one could be hers, until they start to become buildings.

I have existed for 21 years.

I didn't live them all, but from now on I am hoping to.

I take my medication, though one day I want to come off it. Sometimes I have bad days where grey thoughts saunter in like unwanted dinner guests; the trick is not to invite them to sit at the table. They get bored in time, and show themselves out the back door.

Occasionally I hear the ghost of my friend, tumbling down a forgotten corridor.

Let's review that action, She might say. Or, *In the end it is all done.*

Except it's not her, not really. It is only me, the times I get lonely, or fearful, and I try to imagine her back. Something about the voice is off—like an impressionist who's an inch off the mark. I see through it.

I see myself.

I go to my support group. I have proper friends there now, and you can laugh or cry or say nothing at all.

No one minds either way.

I am grateful for the small things: for walking down the street and not being so engulfed in routines I can't see where I'm going.

For having a child sit opposite me on the train and not

worrying which part of their body my eyes alight on.

For every time I enjoy something beautiful, without telling myself that I will focus on it once I have finished my routines.

I can actually follow the plot of TV programs now, and I no longer use books as masks—I read them like a normal person, just like you have read this. Which assumes you are normal; maybe you're not. Maybe none of us are. Maybe none of us would want to be anyway. But, for the sake of argument, let's call me normal now.

I am better. I don't know whether it's for good, or if one day something might make me abnormal again. But that's the funny thing about living. If you do it properly, you don't know how the next sentence will begin.

ABOUT THE AUTHOR

Lily Bailey is a model and writer. Her career in journalism began in 2012, editing a news site and writing about life and fashion for the *Richmond Magazine* and the *Kingston Magazine*. She lives in London.